Rehabilitation Technology

Rehabilitation Technology

Glenn Hedman
Editor

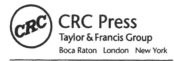

CRC Press
Taylor & Francis Group
Boca Raton   London   New York

CRC Press is an imprint of the
Taylor & Francis Group, an informa business

Rehabilitation Technology has also been published as *Physical & Occupational Therapy in Pediatrics*, Volume 10, Number 2 1990.

Library of Congress Cataloging-in-Publication Data

Rehabilitation technology / Glenn Hedman editor.
    p. cm.
    "Has also been published as Physical & occupational therapy in pediatrics, volume 10, number 2 1990" — T.p. verso.
    Includes bibliographical references.
    ISBN 1-56024-033-4 (acid-free paper)
    1. Physically handicapped children — Rehabilitation — Equipment and supplies. 2. Rehabilitation technology. I. Hedman, Glenn.
    [DNLM: 1. Biomedical Engineering — instrumentation. 2. Rehabilitation — in infancy & childhood. 3. Self-Help Devices. W1 PH683P v. 10 no. 2 / WS 368 R345]
RJ138.R438 1990
617.1'03'083 — dc20
DNLM/DLC
for Library of Congress

90-4593
CIP

This collection is dedicated to the memory of Ron Kett and Sam McFarland, two Rehabilitation Engineers who left us much too soon during 1989. Their good work helped many people and their friendship inspired us to help others.

ABOUT THE EDITOR

Glenn Hedman, MEME, BSBE, is Director of the Assistive Technology Unit of the University of Illinois at Chicago's University Affiliated Program. The center works with clients and their needs in environmental control, computer access, augmentative communication, mobility, seating, and worksite modification. Active in the field of rehabilitation technology for nearly a decade, Mr. Hedman is the past director of the Department of Rehabilitation Engineering at the Rehabilitation Institute of Chicago.

Mr. Hedman received his Bachelor of Science in Bioengineering from the University of Illinois at Chicago and earned his Master of Engineering degree in the Rehabilitation Engineering Graduate Program from the University of Virginia.

Rehabilitation Technology

CONTENTS

Foreword

I have read the articles contributed to this special collection with a great deal of interest. It is pleasing to see an entire collection dedicated to technology in rehabilitation. The use of technology to meet the needs of individuals with disabilities has accelerated each year for the past decade. The role that assistive devices can play in improving the function of a disabled person and augmenting the rehabilitation process has been clearly demonstrated.

It is also particularly exciting to look at the authorship of these articles. The authors are representative of a group of creative and energetic therapists and clinicians who have embraced technology and have made great contributions to the widespread use of assistive devices.

As an engineer, I am interested in the design process. Design can be defined as rigorous engineering design, and also as technical problem solving. I believe that much of rehabilitation technology falls into the problem solving category. While on the faculty at Tufts University, several of my colleagues and I became interested in encouraging nonengineers to participate more formally in the technical problem solving associated with rehabilitation. We developed several courses aimed at enhancing the design skills of clinicians. We were not alone in those efforts. Across the nation clinicians, like the authors of these articles were expanding their horizons.

The interdisciplinary nature of assistive technology is no better illustrated than in the organization known as RESNA. This group was originally established in the late 1970's as the Rehabilitation Engineering Society of North America. It primarily focused on the research and education needs of engineers who were involved in the design, development, and research of new devices in rehabilitation. The focus of RESNA rapidly grew to include the broader issues of service delivery, funding, education, quality assurance, and public policy. As was only natural, the membership expanded not only in numbers, but in disciplines. Today, with over 1200 members, RESNA includes significant numbers of occupational therapists, physical therapists, speech pathologists, physicians, special educators, as well as rehabilitation engineers. Representatives of these varied disciplines come together for a common purpose within RESNA.

I am in the final year of my term as President of RESNA. Interestingly, I have followed two nonengineers who held this office before me. We believe that RESNA is truly an interdisciplinary organization.

Recent federal legislation has focused increased attention on the use of assistive technology. With additional funding being provided for the development of state infrastructures, there will be an increasing need for us to guarantee that technology lives up to its advanced billing. We need to constantly remember that technology alone offers very little. It is the use of technology within a caring society that increases the function of a person with disability. It is the integration of technology into the rehabilitation and education systems that will yield substantial results.

In each of the articles in this special collection, the reader will find several common messages. All of the authors show the use of technology can really make a difference. The examples which they provide, show that appropriate technology can serve as an important part of the rehabilitation process. We should all be encouraged by these successes.

The articles also continually emphasize the need for cooperation among disciplines in order to make the technology work. The articles go beyond the idea of a "team approach" to assistive technology. The team is not just the clinical staff augmented by an engineer. These authors have a clear understanding that we need to make use of all of the resources at hand. The assistive technology team includes the traditional disciplines, the client, the family, the funding source, and the community in which the consumer lives.

Assistive technology does not belong to any specific field or discipline. It cuts across nearly all professions in rehabilitation and special education. It is important that we realize that each of us has a major contribution to make in the successful integration of disabled people into the mainstream of society. Each of us also can make a creative contribution to the use of technology.

Richard Foulds, PhD
President, RESNA
Director, Applied Science and Engineering Laboratories
A.I. duPont Institute
P.O. 269
Wilmington, DE 19899

Preface

As I was compiling this special collection on Rehabilitation Technology, I was concerned that the topic of Rehabilitation Technology might elicit visions of calculators, neatly sharpened number 2 pencils, and pocket liners in the minds of potential readers. Although these *are* functional items, the field contains much, much more.

The topics presented, Seating and Positioning, Powered Mobility, Controls, Computer Access, Prosthetics and Orthotics, and Funding reflect some of the areas of work in Rehabilitation Technology today. A much larger volume would be needed to address all areas of work in the field. Augmentative Communication is purposely excluded since it was the focus of a previous collection of articles (*Physical & Occupational Therapy in Pediatrics*, Volume 7, Number 2). The Appendix contains a listing of references on Funding because of its underlying importance; Rehabilitation Technology must be obtained before its benefits can be realized.

The devices presented are not meant to be a catalog of commercially-available products. Such a book would be soon out-of-date. Instead, we have attempted to first provide a structure of the types of devices in each area, then give a ''snap-shot'' of what devices are used in each area of Rehabilitation Technology today and where they fit into that structure. If we succeed, the reader will be able to better understand the devices that become available in the future and know what qualities they should look for in those devices.

No discussion of Rehabilitation Technology or Rehabilitation Engineering would be complete without reference to the confusing definitions of the terms ''Rehabilitation Technology'' and ''Rehabilitation Engineering.'' Although Rehabilitation Engineering work includes the design and production of devices for persons with disabilities and is an essential component of service delivery, the term

xiii

Rehabilitation Technology more accurately covers the current team-approach focus of service delivery.

I have many people to thank in this endeavor. First, the volume's editors, Suzann Campbell, Ph.D. and Irma Wilhelm, M.S., and The Haworth Press for asking me to put this collection together and for their interest in Rehabilitation Technology. Second, the authors of the chapters for the hard work they put into their manuscripts; these talented people will now be able to answer phone calls and open mail fearlessly for the revisions are over. Third, my friend Lois Deming Hedman, for her encouragement throughout this process.

We all know the precious nature of life. The use of Rehabilitation Technology in helping a child to achieve independence in life can bring great joy.

LET THE FUN BEGIN!!!

Glenn Hedman

Chapter 1

Overview of Rehabilitation Technology

Glenn Hedman

Technology has affected the lives of all people. No population, though, has the potential to benefit from technology more than children with disabilities. Many aspects of a child's life, communication, independent mobility, comfort, safety, and play, for example, are assisted by the existence of technology.[1,2]

The impact of technology on the lives of children with disabilities has occurred in three basic ways: (1) through the infusion of technology into the lives of all people through devices such as remote control appliances; (2) through the development of devices specific to the needs of persons with disabilities such as communication aids, specialized seating, and prostheses; and (3) through the adaptation of devices made for persons without physical disabilities so that they can be used by all people.

Much of the work in the area of Rehabilitation Technology began with the establishment of federally-supported Rehabilitation Engineering Centers in 1972. These centers each focused on a specific area of Rehabilitation Technology. Each Center worked to get the devices it produced into people's lives, through service delivery and/or through having the devices make the transition to the commercial market.

The 1980s produced an emphasis on the delivery of services to

Glenn Hedman, BSBE, MEME, is currently Coordinator, Assistive Technology Unit, University of Illinois at Chicago, 1640 West Roosevelt, Chicago, IL 60608. Prior to his present position, he served as Director of the Rehabilitation Institute of Chicago's Rehabilitation Engineering Department for five years.

1

the consumer. This is reflected in the areas of concentration of the 16 Rehabilitation Engineering Centers identified in 1986 (see Resources listing at the end of this chapter).

The 1980s also brought many advances in legislation as well as technology. Two significant bills, the 1986 Amendments to the Rehabilitation Act (Public Law 99-506) and the 1988 Technology-Related Assistance for Individuals with Disabilities Act (Public Law 100-407) may make Rehabilitation Technology more accessible to those that can benefit from it.

As defined by the 1986 Amendments to the Rehabilitation Act, the term rehabilitation engineering means "the systematic application of technologies, engineering methodologies, or scientific principles to meet the needs of and address the barriers confronted by individuals with handicaps in areas which include education, rehabilitation, employment, transportation, independent living, and recreation."[3] This law has particularly helped to encourage the availability of Rehabilitation Technology services in vocational settings.

The 1988 Technology-Related Assistance for Individuals with Disabilities Act represents a chance for individual states to develop their own state-wide Rehabilitation Technology service delivery systems. The grant competition will allow the chosen states to implement their plans over a three-, four-, or five-year period. Readers are encouraged to contact their representatives in Congress to check the status of the legislation and how it relates to their state.

LOW-TECH vs. HIGH-TECH

The term "high-tech" is joining the overused section of the language inhabited by other terms like "networking." The term "low-tech" has been used to describe devices and modifications which seem to stem from common sense, inexpensive approaches to problem-solving.

Although the use of levers on tape recorder controls to allow operation by a child with a spinal cord injury does not represent a high-tech approach in 1990, use of levers to assist in a task probably would have been considered high-tech a couple of thousand years ago. Since the two terms seem to depend, in part, on the era the particular approach was developed, we will refrain from using the two terms and instead consider all approaches to meeting the needs of persons with disabilities as being part of Rehabilitation Technology.

Although this may seem to be a trivial issue, it is important in that the quality of simplicity is an important goal in meeting the needs of persons with disabilities. Not every problem needs a high-tech solution and those that do usually have a low-tech aspect to them. It is only through the open-minded consideration of all available technology that a successful solution is found. If a particular combination of technological devices has the following qualities, it is a successful solution:

- Solves the problem at hand
- Does not create problems in other areas
- Is obtainable by the client
- Will hold up in the environment in which used
- Is serviceable
- Will meet the client's needs in the reasonable future until another device is appropriate

The number of Rehabilitation Technology devices that are available today is staggering. Yet, few are used "off-the-shelf." Most need some adjustment, training of the user, or have an issue such as attachment to the person's mobility device, that must be addressed. Some may need modification to allow access to the device at all. These examples illustrate the need for the Rehabilitation Technology Team to have the ability to "customize" devices for the consumer.

An economical approach in the application of Rehabilitation Technology can be summarized in the following way:

- First choice: Recommendation of a commercially-available device to address the need.
- Second choice: Modification of a commercially-available device.
- Third choice: Custom-fabrication of a device.

Consumers presented only with a custom-fabricated option as a solution to their problem should be extremely cautious. This option is often the most expensive, takes the longest to produce, and is the most difficult to service. Even custom-fabricated options should have a healthy supply of commercially-available components (for persons with disabilities, for the entire population, or for industry). Mann states that persons with disabilities "are most readily and economically served when devices for their benefit are but modest adaptations of commercially produced, aggressively marketed products purchased by a significant segment of the public."[4]

As the number of devices has grown, efforts have begun to standardize the terminology and characteristics of performance of some. McLaurin has been instrumental in the development of standards for wheelchairs and seating.[6] Efforts in refinement and alternative design of devices such as powered mobility base controllers or keyboard layout are always underway.[7,8,9]

The existence of Rehabilitation Technology "Teams" is an indirect result of the number of devices that are commercially-available. The application of Rehabilitation Technology devices has shifted from the evaluation efforts of research labs to the offices of clinicians where they are recommended as tools to be used by their clients. Consumers coming to Rehabilitation Technology service delivery outlets are tapping into the expertise of the Rehabilitation Technology team professionals to obtain a device or devices, with any necessary modifications, that will successfully meet their needs. The Rehabilitation Technology team members typically can include:[5]

- Client
- Occupational Therapist
- Physical Therapist
- Speech/Language Pathologist
- Rehabilitation Engineer
- Rehabilitation Engineering Technician
- Orthotist
- Prosthetist
- Physician

The particular team members needed will depend on the particular situation at hand.

Rehabilitation Technology Teams exist in numerous settings. A good description of the various sites of application of Rehabilitation Technology is located in the publication Rehabilitation Technology – A Practical Guide.[10] These include:

- Durable Medical Equipment (DME) Supplier
- Department within a Comprehensive Rehabilitation Program
- Technology Service Delivery Center in a University
- State Agency-Based Program
- Private Rehabilitation Engineering/Technology Firm
- Local Affiliate of a National Non-Profit Disability Organization
- Miscellaneous Types of Programs, including Volunteer Groups and Information Resource Centers

Mobile service delivery teams are becoming more common, either used alone or in conjunction with a permanent service delivery office.[11,12] Mobile services can be limited by space and cost restraints, but they are often the most effective means of making Rehabilitation Technology accessible to the public.

The availability of Rehabilitation Technology resources varies a great deal from state to state. As such, no one model of Rehabilitation Technology service delivery can be presented to describe all settings. Clinicians investigating the usefulness of Rehabilitation Technology in addressing their clients' needs will need to tap into whatever resources are available to them. This may include the obtaining of devices manufactured for the entire population available at hardware or electronics stores.

One resource that may be of help is the Rehabilitation Technology Service Delivery Directory (developed by **RESNA, An Interdisciplinary Association for the Advancement of Rehabilitation and Assistive Technologies**; see Resources listing at the end of this chapter). It lists the professionals involved in Rehabilitation Technology in each state and what areas of Rehabilitation Technology they work in. Even if the type of service needed in a given area is not handled by the nearest professional, they may be a good source of information as to where the particular service can be found most readily.

As technology has had an impact on all areas of rehabilitation, many organizations representing consumers and professionals have formed groups to allow their members to keep up with advancements. A listing of organizations appears in the Resources list for those wishing to develop this area of interest.

Two organizations in particular concentrate on Rehabilitation Technology. **RESNA, An Interdisciplinary Association for the Advancement of Rehabilitation and Assistive Technologies**, is an organization comprised of consumers and rehabilitation professionals that deals with the research and service delivery of Rehabilitation Technology. **Closing the Gap** deals with information regarding the application of Rehabilitation Technology in Special Education and Rehabilitation settings.

It is hoped that these organizations can provide a means of keeping their members apprised of new developments as the needs of persons with disabilities are addressed today and in the future.

It is important that Rehabilitation Technology makes its way into the lives of children with disabilities. By doing so, the needs that they have now can be addressed and they can become familiar with the benefits of technology as they face other issues of independence in school settings, the arts, and in vocational endeavors.[13]

REFERENCES

1. Levy R, Cinq-Mars I: A play environment project for children with disabilities, in *Proceedings: 1979 International Conference on Rehabilitation Engineering*, 1979, pp. 1-8.

2. Okumura R: Designing assistive devices for developmental tasks in recreation, in *Proceedings of the Ninth Annual Conference on Rehabilitation Technology*, 1986, pp. 52-54.

3. Enders A: Rehabilitation Act reauthorized for five years. *Rehabilitation Technology Review* 5 (3): 1986.

4. Mann RW: Selective perspectives on a quarter century of rehabilitation engineering. *Journal of Rehabilitation Research and Development* 23 (4): 1-6, 1986.

5. Kohn JG: The physician's role in obtaining rehabilitation technology, in *Proceedings of the 10th Annual Conference on Rehabilitation Technology*, 1987, pp. 356-357.

6. McLaurin C: Wheelchair development, standards, progress, and issues: A

discussion with Colin McLaurin, Sc.D. *Journal of Rehabilitation Research and Development* 23 (2): 48-51, 1986.

7. Riley PO, Rosen MJ: Evaluating manual control devices for those with tremor disability. *Journal of Rehabilitation Research and Development* 24 (2): 99-110, 1987.

8. Brown KE, Inigo RM, Johnson BW: An adaptable optimal controller for electric wheelchairs. *Journal of Rehabilitation Research and Development* 24 (2): 87-98, 1987.

9. Chubon RA, Hester MR: An enhanced standard computer keyboard system for single-finger and typing-stick typing. *Journal of Rehabilitation Research and Development* 25 (4): 17-24, 1988.

10. Smith RO: Models of service delivery in rehabilitation technology, in *Rehabilitation Technology Service Delivery: A Practical Guide*. Washington, DC, RESNA, 1987, pp. 7-25.

11. Law DF, Schuch J: The nation's first mobile rehabilitation engineering unit, in *Proceedings of the Eighth Annual Conference on Rehabilitation Technology*, 1985, pp. 189-190.

12. Dodds R: Rehabilitation technology services: A mobile rehabilitation engineering department, in *Proceedings of the 10th Annual Conference on Rehabilitation Technology*, 1987, pp. 13-14.

13. Charles D, James KB, Stein RB: Rehabilitation of musicians with upper limb amputations. *Journal of Rehabilitation Research and Development* 25 (3): 25-32, 1988.

RESOURCES

REHABILITATION ENGINEERING CENTERS (RECS):

Center for Rehabilitation Technology Services, South Carolina Vocational Rehabilitation Department, 1410-C Boston Avenue, P.O. Box 15, West Columbia, SC 29171-0015, (803) 739-5362

Connecticut's REC, Institute for Human Resource Development, 78 Eastern Boulevard, Glastonbury, CT 06033, (203) 659-1166

Harvard-MIT REC, Massachusetts Institute of Technology, 77 Massachusetts Avenue, Building 3, Room 137, Cambridge, MA 02139

REC on Access to Computers and Electronic Equipment, University of Wisconsin-Madison Trace Center, 1500 Highland Avenue, Madison, WI 53705

REC on Augmentative Communication, University of Delaware / A.I. Dupont Institute, Applied Science and Engineering Laboratory, P.O. Box 269, Wilmington, DE 19899, (302) 651-6830

REC for Development and Evaluation of Sensory Aids for Blind, Visually Impaired, and Deaf-Blind Individuals, Smith-Kettlewell Eye Research Institute, 2232 Webster Street, San Francisco, CA 94115, (415) 561-1630

REC on Evaluation of Rehabilitation Technology, National Rehabilitation

Hospital, Rehabilitation Engineering Services, 102 Irving Street, NW, Washington, DC 20010, (202) 877-1932, (202) 726-3996 (TDDC)

REC on Functional Electrical Stimulation for Restoration of Neural Control, Case Western Reserve University, Cleveland Metropolitan General Hospital, 3395 Scranton Road, Cleveland, OH 44109, (216) 459-3480

REC on Improved Wheelchair and Seating Design, University of Virginia, Box 3368 — University Station, Charlottesville, VA 22903, (804) 977-6730

REC on Modifications to Worksites and Educational Settings, CP Research Foundation of Kansas, Inc., 2021 North Old Manor, Box 8217, Wichita, KS 67208 (316) 688-1888

REC in Prosthetics and Orthotics, Northwestern University Rehabilitation Engineering Program, 345 East Superior Street — Room 1441, Chicago, IL 60611, (312) 908-8560

REC for Quantification of Human Performance, Ohio State University, 471 Dodd Drive, Columbus, OH 43210, (614) 293-3808

REC on Rehabilitation Technology Transfer, Professional Staff Association, Rancho Los Amigos Medical Center, Inc., 7601 East Imperial Highway, Bonita Hall, Downey, CA 90242, (213) 940-7994

REC on Rehabilitation Technology Transfer, Electronic Industries Foundation, 1901 Pennsylvania Avenue, NW, Suite 700, Washington, DC 20006, (202) 955-5823

REC on Technological Aids for Deaf and Hearing Impaired Individuals, The Lexington Center, Inc., Research and Training Division, 30th Avenue and 75th Street, Jackson Heights, NY 11370, (718) 899-8800, ext 333

Vermont REC for Low Back Pain, University of Vermont, 1 South Prospect Street, Burlington, VT 05401, (802) 656-4582, (800) LBP-7320

PUBLICATIONS

Directory of National Information Sources on Handicapping Conditions and Related Services, National Institute on Disability and Rehabilitation Research, U.S. Department of Education, Office of Special Education and Rehabilitative Services, Mary Switzer Building, 330 C Street, SW, Washington, DC 20202, (202) 732-1186

Technology for Independent Living Sourcebook, Alexandra Enders, Editor, Available from RESNA (see below)

ORGANIZATIONS

ABLENET, Cerebral Palsy Center, Griggs-Midway Building, 1821 University Avenue, St. Paul, MN 55104, (612) 331-5958

ALEXANDER GRAHAM BELL ASSOCIATION FOR THE DEAF, 3417 Volta Place, Washington, DC 20007, (202) 337-5220 (Voice/TDD)

AMERICAN COUNCIL FOR THE BLIND (ACB), Suite 100, 1010 Vermont Avenue, NW, Washington, DC 20005, (202) 393-3666, (800) 424-8666

AMERICAN FOUNDATION FOR THE BLIND, 15 West 16th Street, New York, NY 10011, (212) 620-2000

AMERICAN OCCUPATIONAL THERAPY ASSOCIATION (AOTA), 1383 Piccard Drive, Rockville, MD 20850, (301) 948-9626

AMERICAN ORTHOTIC AND PROSTHETIC ASSOCIATION (AOPA), 717 Pendleton Street, Alexandria, VA 22314, (703) 836-7116

AMERICAN PHYSICAL THERAPY ASSOCIATION (APTA), 111 North Fairfax Street, Alexandria, VA 22314, (703) 684-2782

AMERICAN SPEECH-LANGUAGE-HEARING ASSOCIATION (ASHA), 10801 Rockville Pike, Rockville, MD 20852, (301) 897-5700 (Voice/TDD)

ASSOCIATION FOR CHILDREN AND ADULTS WITH LEARNING DISABILITIES (ACLD), 4156 Library Road, Pittsburgh, PA 15234, (412) 341-1515, (412) 341-8077

CENTER FOR SPECIAL EDUCATION TECHNOLOGY, 1920 Association Drive, Reston, VA 22091, (703) 620-3660, (800) 345-TECH (Limited hours)

CLOSING THE GAP, P.O. Box 68, Henderson, MN 56044, (612) 248-3294

CONGRESS OF ORGANIZATIONS OF THE PHYSICALLY HANDICAPPED (COPH), 16630 Beverly Avenue, Tinley Park, IL 60477, (312) 532-3566

MUSCULAR DYSTROPHY ASSOCIATION (MDA), 810 Seventh Avenue, New York, NY 10019, (212) 586-0808

NATIONAL ASSOCIATION FOR THE DEAF (NAD), 814 Thayer Avenue, Silver Spring, MD 20910, (301) 587-1788 (Voice/TDD)

NATIONAL EASTER SEAL SOCIETY, 70 East Lake Street, Chicago, IL 60601, (312) 726-6200

NATIONAL FEDERATION OF THE BLIND (NFB), 1800 Johnson Street, Baltimore, MD 21230, (301) 659-9314

NATIONAL HEAD INJURY FOUNDATION, 333 Turnpike Road, Southborough, MA 01772, (508) 485-9950

NATIONAL INFORMATION CENTER FOR DEAFNESS (NICD), Gallaudet University, 800 Florida Avenue, NE, Washington, DC 20002, (202) 651-5051 (Voice), (202) 651-5052 (TDD)

NATIONAL MULTIPLE SCLEROSIS SOCIETY, 205 East 42nd Street, New York, NY 10017, (212) 986-3240

RESNA — An Association for the Advancement of Rehabilitation Technology, Suite 700, 1101 Connecticut Avenue, N.W., Washington, D.C. 20036, (202) 857-1199, (202) 775-2625 (FAX)

SELF HELP FOR HARD OF HEARING PEOPLE (SHHH), 7800 Wisconsin Avenue, Bethesda, MD 20814, (301) 657-2248 (Voice), (301) 657-2249 (TDD)

UNITED CEREBRAL PALSY ASSOCIATIONS (UCPA), 66 East 34th Street, New York, NY 10016, (212) 481-6300

Sources include:

Trachtman, L: Technology Resources Nationally. Presented at *Role of Technology in Successful Placement of the Disabled Client.* Rehabilitation Institute of

Chicago, Department of Education and Training. Chicago, IL. August 24-25, 1989.

Directory of National Information Sources on Handicapping Conditions and Related Services. See "Publications."

Rehab/Education Technology Resourcebook Series: Communication, Control, and Computer Access for Disabled and Elderly Individuals, by Trace Research and Development Center. Boston: College-Hill Press.

Enders, A: *Assistive Technology Sourcebook*, RESNA, 1989.

Chapter 2

Seating Systems:
The Therapist and Rehabilitation
Engineering Team

Jessica Presperin

Not long ago, a therapist, wishing to order a wheelchair, merely made a selection from one or two catalogs and decided among a few options. The influence of rehabilitation technology on the world of seating and positioning has inundated the market with a vast selection of mobility bases (wheelchairs) and positioning equipment. Even with all the adaptive equipment that is available, however, there is still a need for custom fabrication.

Adrienne Bergen, PT, Joan Bergmann, PT, Cheryl Colangelo, OTR, and Elaine Trefler, OTR, are therapists who pioneered in the area of seating and positioning. Their input on assessment methods, measurements, and system recommendations provided the basis for positioning today. Although their work mainly focused on children with central nervous system (CNS) deficits, many of the theoretical concepts apply to adult and geriatric clients as well. This article will not cover the criteria for assessment and measurement of a client requiring a seating system. Those clinicians interested in seriously

Jessica Presperin provides consultation services in Occupational Therapy, specifically regarding Seating and Positioning, in San Diego, CA. She has lectured extensively in the United States and Europe on these topics.

The author would like to thank Cathy Bazata, OTR/L and BJ Jenkins, PT, for their editorial input. Thanks are expressed to Bill Walker, Bill Conyers, and C. Kerry Jones, RE, formerly of the Rehab. Technology Center in South Bend, IN for their engineering expertise in the fabrication of many of the systems described.

pursuing development of these skills can refer to the resources provided at the end of this chapter.[1-4] One should note that there are no "cookbook" answers to seating. Theoretical implications, although justified in the literature, may not always hold true in the clinical setting.

Clinicians began by observing that the vinyl of most wheelchairs would eventually sling and cause a hammock-like surface. This promoted a posterior pelvic tilt, adduction and internal rotation of the lower extremities, and kyphosis of the trunk.[1] Following this observation, therapists began providing a firm seat and back surface. At the onset of this type of intervention, those interested in providing postural support began using materials such as triwall, ethafoam, plywood, and anything commercially available to meet the clients needs.[5] (See Figure 1.)

Clinical observation of the individual before and after technologi-

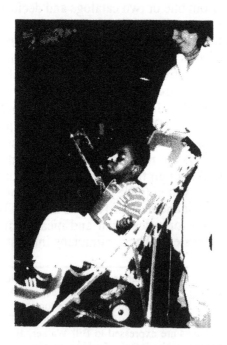

FIGURE 1. Tri-wall insert in stroller with hip guides, trunk supports, and head roll.

cal intervention showed dramatic changes, not only in the postural and cosmetic appearance but functionally and medically as well. It has been documented that seating and positioning can have a direct correlation with the prevention of pressure sores, orthopedic deformities, and muscle contractures as well as with qualitative improvements in respiration, digestion, heart rate, and functional skills.[1,2,4,6,7]

Clinicians began to view seating and positioning as an adjunct to therapy, often enhancing the attainment of a functional goal. Improvement of seating and positioning has become an acceptable objective for goal setting in a therapist's treatment plan. As therapists began to study the impact of proper positioning on the client's body, more sophisticated ideas were formulated. The field of rehabilitation engineering had much to offer in these endeavors. The skills of the rehabilitation engineer paired with a therapist specialized in seating and positioning allow for evaluation, simulation, recommendation and, if necessary, fabrication and/or modification of an optimal positioning device for each client.

SIMULATION

Saftler, Waugh, and Winters,[8] were key physical therapists in demonstrating the need for simulation to determine optimal positioning. In the Florida state-funded, "Therapeutic Equipment Specialist" courses, taught in the early 1980s to the present, instructors presented the technique of taking measurements and using a specially designed simulator to determine the optimal seated position for the client. The simulator allowed the therapist to try various angles, including seat-to-back, seat-to-calf, and calf-to-foot. Leg length, seat depth, medial or lateral thigh supports, back height, trunk supports, head supports, arm rest devices and angle of tilt, all could be evaluated for the client. Planar (flat) and contoured (specifically curved to the client's body) approaches also could be simulated (see Figures 2-11). In their work, joined later by Cathy Bazata, OTR and BJ Jenkins, PT, they were able to determine the client's best position for sitting tolerance, weight distribution, and functional capabilities. The simulations also allowed observation of the client's tonal and behavioral response to position changes and the effect of stabilizing forces on the body. Theoretical concepts do not always hold true in a real-life setting. A thorough simulation, followed by the taking of exact measurements, saved time on revisions caused by ill-fittings and the erroneous decisions made frequently without simulation.[9] Support systems and angles often have to be changed to accommodate the effects on the client. Today, several seating centers, rehabilitation equipment dealers, and seating specialists use simulators to determine optimal seating components for their clients. Some institutions have fabricated their own simulators, allowing them to mock up components used most frequently in their centers. Hopital Marie Enfant in Montreal, Rehabilitation Technology Center in Indianapolis, University of Iowa in Iowa City, and IWK Children's Hospital in New Brunswick have used their own simulators extensively with success.

Two simulators are now commercially available: The Flamingo from Tallahassee Therapeutics (see Figure 2), and the KISS from Pin Dot Products (see Figure 3). Both offer options for planar and contour simulation as well as componentry and the ability to assess powered mobility. Besides the time saved and ability to assess the impact of the intervention, the clinician can take pictures of the client in their present system followed by one in the simulator. These pictures demonstrate the justification of recommended equipment to the physician and third party reimbursement agencies.[10]

PLANAR vs. CONTOUR

As noted above, therapists now have the option of choosing planar or contoured systems. A planar system is generally flat, although generic curves used in the "contour gauge back," described later, may be classified as planar. Because planar components do not follow the specific contours of the body, they allow the system to grow with the individual. Supports can be moved higher and wider as the individual changes. A disadvantage is that sacral and lateral support provided by a more intimate fit may be sacrificed (see Figures 4, 5, and 6).

Once thought of as an expensive luxury, the contoured system has proven its worth in the world of seating and positioning.[11] Many

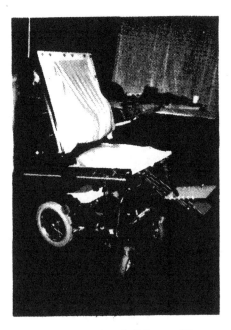

FIGURE 2. The Flamingo (Tallahassee Therapeutics).

contoured systems are in the same price range today as planar systems. The contoured system was originally designed for the severely involved client with multiple orthopedic deformities. The contours allow closer body contact, improving the pressure distribution while providing needed support. It was later found that contours, especially in the sacral and trunk area, provide excellent support for hypotonic individuals lacking the musculature to tolerate upright sitting.[11,12,13,14]

Contoured systems do not necessarily have to be "glove fitting." They can be molded to provide support while allowing growth and some active movement. Contoured systems can be (1) poured around the body using a liquid chemical mixture that hardens into different densities of foam (see Foam-in-Place: Figure 7), (2) molded using a dylantin vacuum consolidation process (see Desemo: Figure 8; Bead Seat: Figures 9a & 9b; Contour-U: Figure 10), (3) high-temperature plastic formed from plaster casts (see Gil-

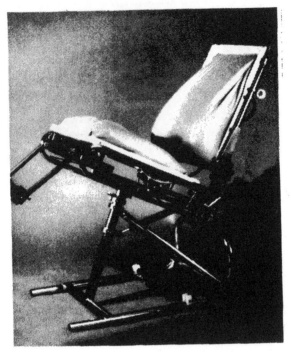

FIGURE 3. The KISS (Pin Dot Products).

lette: Figure 11), (4) carved Ethafoam, or other carved foams.[13,14,15,16,18] Planar and contoured systems are both widely used for seating intervention. The therapists must decide what their goals are for positioning each client and recommend the most optimal cost-effective system to meet that client's needs.

VARIATIONS IN SEATING BY DIAGNOSIS

Although the criteria for assessment and measurement-taking apply across diagnoses, goals may differ, depending on the client's particular physical, cognitive, and behavioral characteristics. Hobson attempted to formulate a general but not exclusive classification system for determining seating options.[15] The three tracts he describes are: "(a) seating for postural control and deformity manage-

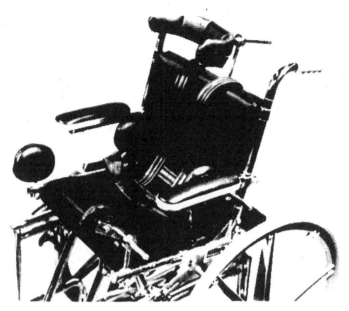

FIGURE 4. Miller Seating System—illustrates flat planar system incorporating lateral knee blocks, trunk supports, headrest, and vest.

ment (Cerebral Palsy population); (b) seating for pressure and postural management (Spinal cord-Injured population); (c) seating for comfort and postural accommodation (Multiply Handicapped and Geriatric populations)."[15] These classifications are not meant to be rigid, because, in some instances, clients may overlap tracts, requiring postural control for one body part and accommodation for another. The goal of forming classifications, however, is to allow the clinician to group clients with similar deficits together in order to prioritize their needs and technological intervention.

(a) Postural Control and Deformity Management

The largest population served by seating centers throughout the country is that of individuals diagnosed with central nervous system deficits such as cerebral palsy, head injury, or stroke. The client with reducible deformities generally falls into this category. As stated before, early intervention using proper seating and position-

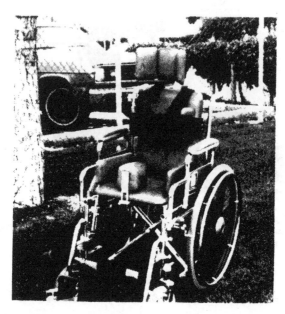

FIGURE 5. Scott Therapeutics System incorporating lateral trunk supports, lateral and medial thigh supports, and headrest.

ing components demonstrates many long term benefits.[1,2,4,7] These benefits include alignment of the skeleton, reduction of tonal influences on the body, stabilization of the pelvis posteriorly and laterally, and increased tolerance of the seated position. Specialists in the field who have been providing intervention to clients at a young age are noting a decrease in the formation of poor habitual motor patterns which lead to deformity, decreased incidents of pressure problems from excessive leaning to one side, decreases in the usual need for surgical intervention, and greater functional capabilities lasting into adolescence and adulthood. The goals for the clinician and engineer working with a client falling into this classification category are to evaluate the client to determine how intervention can influence posture or tonal influences and to select the componentry to do so. The focus is to enable the client to be in a position of "readiness" to promote their highest level of function.[11] Functional activities can range from performing a work-related task using both arms, to using a head pointer for communication, to

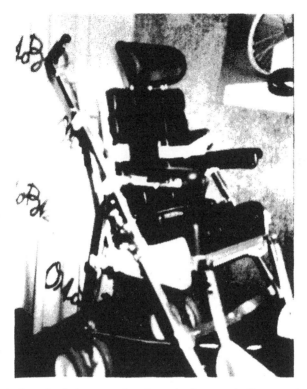

FIGURE 6. Otto Bock System with planar back, generically curved seat, trunk supports, headrest, foot support, and armrests in stroller.

visual tracking. Intervention to prevent the influence of an abnormal reflex or poor posturing without compromising comfort or function of the individual is one of the end goals of the rehabilitation technology team. Intervention may be as simple as providing a firm back and seat, or may require the incorporation of a multitude of components and custom fabrication (see Figures 12, 13a and 13b).

One generally begins seating intervention at the pelvis, providing stability proximally, before continuing with the rest of the body. Clinicians have noted, however, that if an individual demonstrates a strong asymmetrical tonic neck reflex (ATNR) or tonal influence at the head, intervention should begin there. Bergen decreases the in-

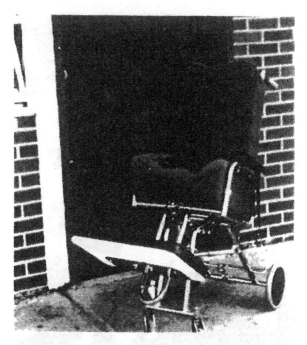

FIGURE 7. Upholstered Foam-in-Place Seating System placed in Safety Travel Chair (photo by Kathy Riley, PT).

fluence of an ATNR by using a head support that places the child's head in a neutral position.[11] As she focuses her initial input on positioning the head, attempting to inhibit the ATNR, she is able to determine other seating components she will need to maintain this desired position. If the influence of the ATNR can be reduced, the potential for asymmetrical deformities appearing later in life is also decreased. A commercialized headrest may not be adequate support for this intricate position. A customized headrest may be required to provide the occipital as well as lateral and anterior support needed at the head. As the clinician provides input for therapeutic placement of the head, the engineer must use his or her knowledge of physics, materials, design, and fabrication. These skills allow the creation of a functional, easy-to-use head piece that is safe, cosmetically acceptable, and durable enough to block the tonal influence as well as endure the repeated handling of the caretakers.

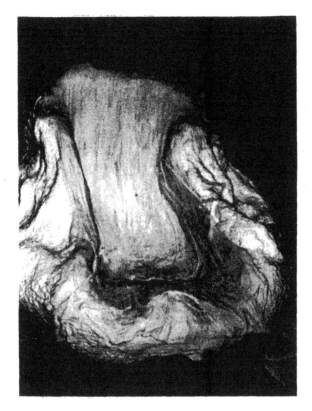

FIGURE 8. The DESEMO System was the first dylantin bag system, developed at the University of Alabama in Birmingham.

Individuals recovering from traumatic head injury also benefit from early assessment and input on seating and positioning needs. Hedman illustrates a series of adjustable seating components used with the head-injured population as they progress through recovery stages.[17,18] By providing immediate positioning capabilities during the rehabilitation stage, the client is able to attend different therapies in an optimal position, and the tonal influences on the body can be reduced, decreasing the potential for poor habit-forming movements and posture. Hedman illustrates the use of flat and generically contoured systems used during the client's rehabilitation stay. An exaggerated anti-thrust seat may be used initially to stabilize a client's pelvis and decrease the influence of a pelvic extensor thrust (see Figure 14). As tone becomes inhibited through time and therapeutic intervention, the severity of the antithrust seat can be reduced to meet the client's needs. The seating system may be tilted back and incorporate the use of trunk supports, lateral and medial thigh

FIGURES 9a and 9b. The Bead Seat System was developed at the University of Tennessee. It allows simulated and actual molding, fabrication, and finishing in one day. ABS plastic modules and hardware allow the system to be formed in the individual's own wheelchair.

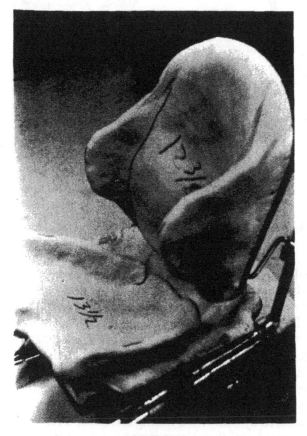

FIGURE 9a

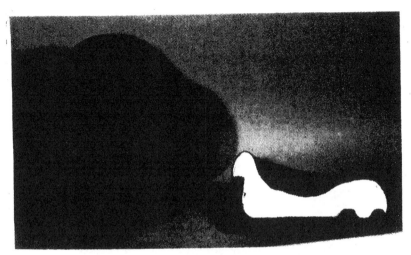

FIGURE 9b

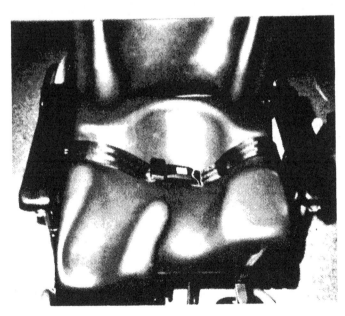

FIGURE 10. The Contour-U System (Pin Dot Products) is a centralized process where plaster molds are taken from the simulator frame and sent to the manufacturer to be made into cushions.

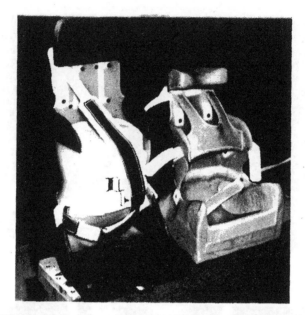

FIGURE 11. Plastic seating systems formed over plaster casts.

supports, headrests and anterior supports. As the client changes in alertness and function, the components can be changed or eliminated. The components can also be interchanged with each other to allow for a variety of different positioning set ups (see Figure 15).

An example of technological input leading to increased function is depicted in the following case study:

A 12-year-old girl suffered a closed head injury resulting in diffuse brain damage. After months of therapy, the client was discharged to home in a standard wheelchair. She had cognitive recovery to the alert-oriented stage. Physically, she had poor balance and minimal lower extremity control. Walking was not considered to be a goal. Both her upper extremities demonstrated severe athetosis. Her left arm exhibited involuntary flailing, causing the client to hit herself in the face, knock her glasses off, or accidentally push things off the table. When asked to perform a functional activity with this hand, the un-

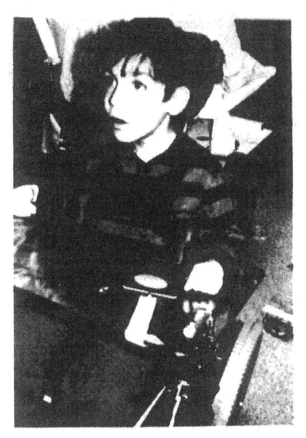

FIGURE 12. The individual is in a planar system consisting of a Jay cushion on a solid base, generically curved back, trunk supports, headrest, positioning vest, and laptray for upper extremity support. The goal was to provide symmetrical support for upright seating, posterior occipital head support with lateral blocks for assisting with head control. Stabilization was gained with the trunk supports, cupping of the pelvis from the cushion, positioning vest, and seat belt. Upper extremity control was enhanced encouraging independence in powered mobility.

controlled movements were exacerbated. The right upper extremity showed no flailing, however, fine motor coordination was impaired. The goal of increasing fine motor coordination and continued therapy for fine motor activities using both extremities appeared futile and humiliating for the client.

When working with the client, the therapist began to assess the client's reactions to increased stabilization. The client was wheeled up to a table and her left arm was placed on the table in a comfortable position of flexion and slight internal rotation. When her arm was held down, the rotational movement of the shoulder girdle and trunk decreased, allowing the client to center herself in the wheelchair. Although the tone fluctuations of the arm were still occurring, the stabilizing force kept the arm on the table and would not allow the arm to move. The client was then able to focus on use of her right arm. When asked to perform tasks using her right arm to place pegs, pick up a filled glass of water, or make x's with a pen, the client

FIGURES 13a and 13b. A contoured seat stabilized the pelvis and prevented an extensor thrust, while a planar bi-angular back (Rehab Designs) provided posterior support and encouraged spinal extension. Components included adjustable trunk supports, shoulder stablizers, foot positioners, and a rolled headrest with lateral temporal supports.

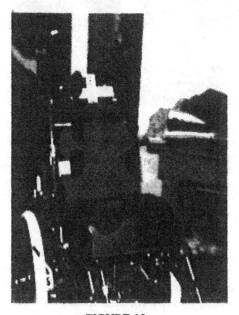

FIGURE 13a

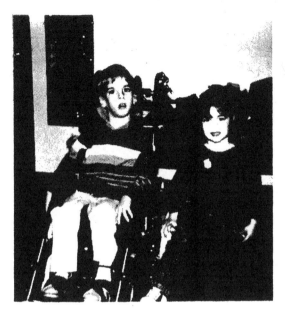

FIGURE 13b

was able to do so with smooth movements. The therapist con-
cluded that stabilization of the client's left arm would reduce
the flailing movements, decrease the influence of these movements on the trunk and allow for increased stability and fine
motor coordination of the opposite extremity.

It is at this time that the rehabilitation engineer was con-
sulted. The solution was to create an upper extremity positioning device. The therapist relayed the clinical situation to the
engineer, demonstrating how she was stabilizing the extremity
and describing the functional capabilities she sought for the
client. The therapist wanted to stabilize the left arm, but allow
the client to be able to use her left hand as an active assist to
hold objects. The engineer's role was to modify a school type
armboard which slides onto the left armrest (see Figure 16).
Stabilizing forces had to be designed and placed on the armrest
that would prevent internal/external rotation, flexion/exten-
sion, and elevation of the shoulder. It had to be strong, dura-

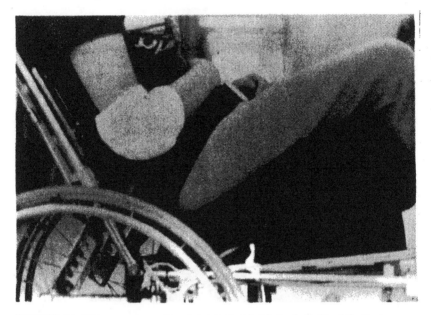

FIGURE 14. This exaggerated anti-thrust seat held the individual in flexion preventing the influence of extensor tone from allowing the client to thrust out of the seating system.

ble, comfortable, easy to use, and cosmetically acceptable to the client. The engineer and therapist worked together to select the best placement for the arm stabilizers. The engineer designed the positioning device using three stabilizers fabricated out of padded ABS plastic and bolted onto the armboard. Velcro straps were then used to hold the arm against these stabilizers. Extraneous movement of the left upper extremity was blocked, allowing the client to stabilize her trunk and gain function of the right upper extremity. The improved fine motor coordination of the client's right arm allowed her to eat and drink without spillage. Along with increased functional skills, the client's dignity was also enhanced. She was no longer embarrassed by involuntary flailing movements and could present herself as a controlled individual in social settings.

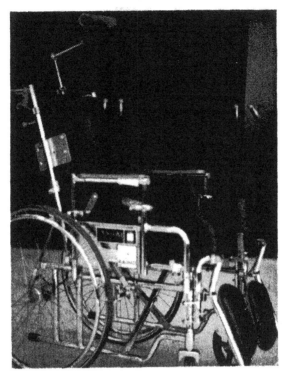

FIGURE 15. RIC adjustable seating system.

(b) Pressure Distribution and Postural Control

Because of decreased or absent sensation, the spinal cord-injured population has an increased need for equalizing pressure distribution. Many cushions are available on the market that decrease the loading on the ischial tuberosities, coccyx, and trochanters. Each client sits differently because of individual differences in body weight and fat distribution. A specific cushion may work for one client and not another. The clinician must assess whether the cushion is, indeed, providing equal pressure distribution. Studies are underway (Helen Hayes Hospital, Sharp Rehab Physical Therapy Dept., and RTC of Memorial Hospital in South Bend) to compare

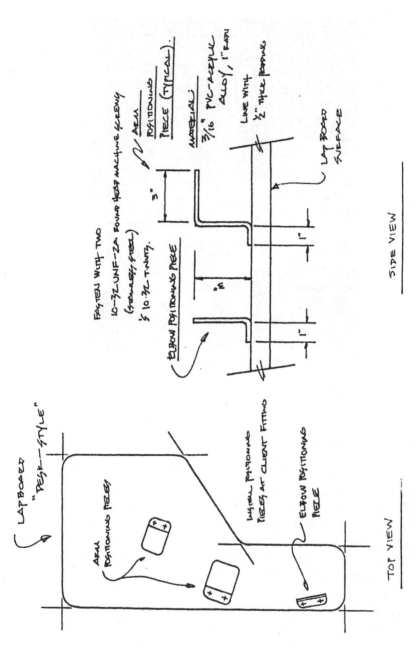

FIGURE 16. Engineering drawing of upper extremity positioner.

commercially available cushions with various clients in different sitting positions. The results of these studies should assist therapists as they work with the client in choosing an appropriate cushion.

Postural stability of the spinal cord-injured (SCI) client is often neglected when deciding on a mobility base and cushion. Individuals with a SCI post five or six years often complain of low back pain.[19,20] Zacharkow[21] notes that the pain is due in part to the prolonged periods of lumbar kyphosis from sitting in the wheelchair. He also states that "shearing force on the buttocks from sitting postures without proper pelvic and sacral support is the most overlooked factor in the etiology of pressure sores." Zacharkow recommends that the seat and back should be reclined to prevent sliding forward, obtain proper trunk stabilization, and keep the individual's back against the backrest.

During 1986-87, Jones (a rehabilitation engineer), Bazata and Presperin (occupational therapists) worked with SCI clients who averaged 4-9 years post injury at the Rehabilitation Technology Center (RTC) in South Bend, Indiana. Although several different types of seating systems were recommended depending on level of injury, function, orthopedic involvement, and mobility, two types of backs were used frequently. One was a generically curved "contoured gauge" back and the other was custom molded to the client.[19] The "contoured gauge" back gently curved around the trunk which provided lateral stabilization of the trunk and midline centering into the positioning system. Sacral/lumbar support was sometimes incorporated into the back if pelvic mobility was sufficient. Scapular cutouts were provided in the back to allow upper extremity movement and "hooking" (see Figures 17a, 17b, 18a, 18b, and 18c). Zacharkow,[21] Minkel,[20] and Krapfl,[22] agree with this focus on seating the population with SCI in their documentation and clinical practices. Minkel states that flat solid backs "do not allow the compensatory posterior shifting of the center of gravity quads need for stability and function. . . . The contour, especially when combined with some tip in space, provides postural alignment."[20] Zacharkow demonstrates that the scapular cutouts not only allow for free arm mobility but also avoid pressure over the outer scapulae and shoulders (see Figure 19).[21] The cushions used in the above situation were fabricated by the engineering team previously working at the

Rehabilitation Technology Center in South Bend. Commercially available backs, similar to the "contoured-gauge," although not incorporating the scapular cut-outs, are available through Jay Products and Luxury Liners. The clinician must take care to make sure the cushion does not push the client too far forward, decreasing the functional ability to push the wheels or balance over the wheelchair frame. Weight of the cushion is also critical for the client doing their own disassembly of the wheelchair. The LaBac power recliner wheelchair incorporates a generic curve into its back and will provide scapular cutouts upon request with an additional charge.

A second back cushion provided was custom contoured to the clients pelvis, sacrum, and back. It provided added sacral support which created an increase in spinal extension by encouraging complete coupling of the vertebrae.[19] This prevented the pelvis from shifting into a posterior pelvic tilt with subsequent kyphotic postur-

FIGURES 17a and 17b. Generically-curved back may support trunk to mid-thoracic region decreasing the need for trunk supports.

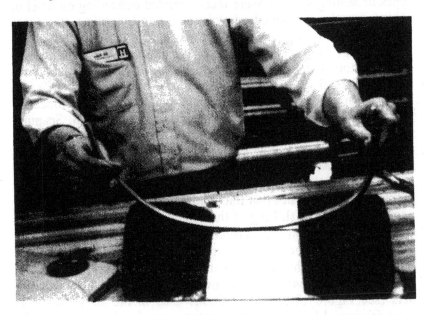

FIGURE 17a

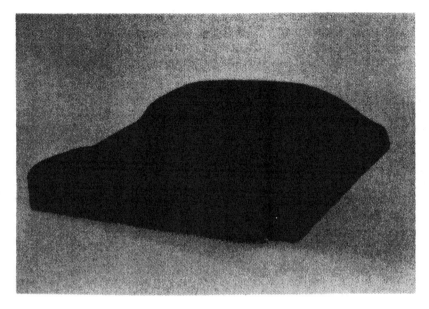

FIGURE 17b

ing. Trunk supports were included as part of the molded back cushion to prevent excessive lateral trunk flexion and to provide the feeling of stability. Relief for the scapulae was also formed into the mold. The seat and back were tilted back slightly (10-15°) to adjust for the change in the client's center of gravity produced by the pelvis being shifted to a neutral or anterior tilt position.

In both situations, a commercially available pressure-reducing cushion was placed on a firm support surface. If the client required greater pelvic stabilization than was provided with a standard cushion, customization was provided. Jay in a Box (Jay Co.) fabricates components which assist in slight stabilization of the pelvis and thighs. ROHO designs a contoured cushion, the Enhancer, which stabilizes the pelvis and channels the legs using variable height bulbs.[23] A contoured cushion can be foamed or molded to provide added control if pressure-reducing foam, gel, flolite, or air bulbs are part of the system. CAD/CAM cushions, presently under study at the University of Virginia, Cleveland Clinic, and Center for

FIGURES 18a, 18b, and 18c. Scapular cutouts as demonstrated below allow free movement of the scapulae for upper extremity movement.

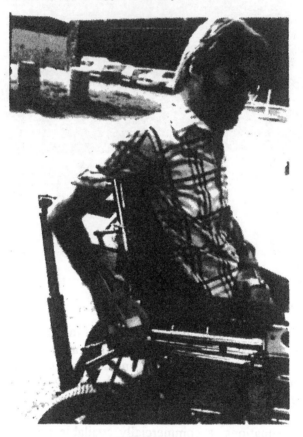

FIGURE 18a

Studies in Aging in Canada, will bring about the ability to fabricate custom-contoured cushions designed to provide pelvic stability as well as pressure reduction.[24,25,26]

Over 60% of the SCI systems designed at RTC, in South Bend were considered to be successful with minimal adaptations provided to the system during follow-up. Most of the clients liked their appearance in the system. Pelvic support provided increased extension of the spine, giving the appearance of increased height. The

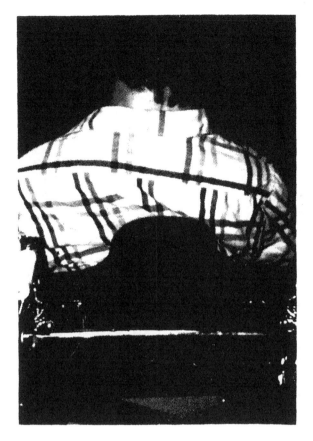

FIGURE 18b

pouched abdomen frequently noted in individuals with SCI was also decreased; however, approximately 35% of the clients were unable to tolerate the position change due to functional or psychological reasons. Functionally, some of the clients were unable to break habitual movement patterns they had developed through the years. The pelvic and spinal extension changes necessitated reaching and moving differently. In many cases, the client believed it was not worth relearning functional patterns over again. Psychologically, because of the change in center of gravity, some clients had the sensation that they were falling forward. They were reluctant to

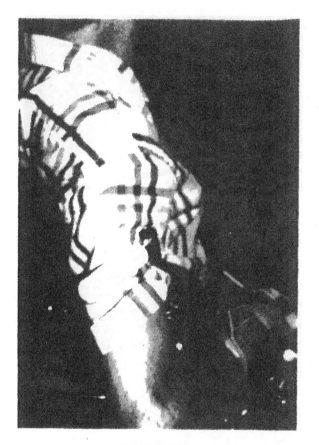

FIGURE 18c

reach out for fear that they would fall. These clients opted to return to the hammocked back system. All clients chose to keep the firm support surface under their pressure-reducing cushions.

Some clients could not use the above back designs because of permanent fixation of their pelvis and spine. These clients were provided "accommodation" systems, which stressed comfort, increased seating tolerance, and improved pressure distribution. The author strongly agrees with Zacharkow, Krapfl, Minkel, and Jones that it is imperative that positioning be done during the initial rehab stages of the client with SCI. This will encourage optimally correct

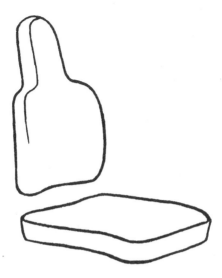

FIGURE 19. A high backrest contoured around the shoulder blades to allow free arm mobility. (Photo from *Posture: Sitting, Standing, Chair Design, and Exercise* by Dennis Zacharkow, courtesy of Charles C Thomas, Publisher, Springfield, Illinois.)

posturing, decrease poor habitual patterning such as hooking, and promote proper weight distribution. The long-term goal is to prevent the predominance of fixed posterior pelvic tilt with resulting kyphotic posture and the incidence of low back pain or pressure sores.

(c) Accommodation

The client with severe non-reducible deformities, regardless of disability, requires a seating system which conforms to his or her body. In most cases the only correction that can be provided for the client is through surgery. Clients falling into this category are older children with cerebral palsy, the multiply handicapped individual, or a geriatric client with fixed deformities. Some of the goals of the seating system are to prevent further deformity, protect the organs from being crushed or moved by the deformed thorax or pelvis, evenly distribute pressure, and provide increased sitting tolerance (see Figures 20a & 20b). In many instances, a contoured seating system is the system of choice; however, clients may be comfortably positioned in planar systems as well.

The therapist must determine the position that (1) the client can tolerate for a period of time, (2) promotes an optimal physiological status and alertness, and (3) encourages functional capabilities. The

FIGURES 20a and 20b. This young teenager demonstrated fixed deformities. Cushions were fabricated to conform to his deformities allowing him to tolerate upright sitting for attendance in day program.

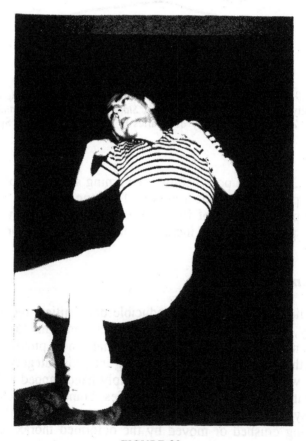

FIGURE 20a

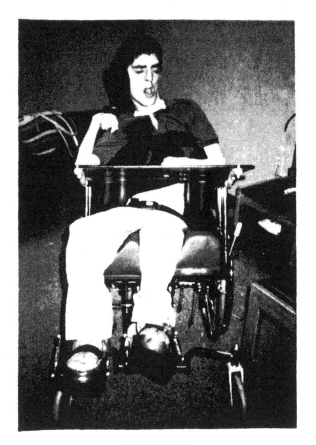

FIGURE 20b

therapist may not be able to change the client's posture, but may wish to place the client in a position where they can function optimally. This may mean allowing the lower extremities to be swept to one side in an effort to promote forward orientation of the shoulders and head. The engineer uses his or her skills to assure that forces supporting the body are strong yet provide maximum comfort and pressure distribution.

Late stage muscular dystrophy (MD) may also fall into the category of accommodation. Previously, clinicians would attempt to support the collapsing spine by incorporating lordosis into the back.

The client would be held in spinal extension with the goal of locking the vertebral facets to discourage spinal rotation and lateral flexion.[27] This approach was unsuccessful and the delay of spinal deformity was minimal. The client's functional capabilities while being forced into this position were compromised.[28] The gravitation pull on the upper extremities while the client was held in extension was too strong, decreasing the individual's ability to use their arms functionally.

The present approach is to perform early surgical procedures to stabilize the spine along with the intervention of proper mobility and seating. Research has demonstrated that this approach has a positive influence on respiratory capabilities of the child with MD.[4,28]

When this procedure has not been used or when the client with MD demonstrates kyphotic positioning and a collapsed trunk, the goal is to accommodate the client for function and comfort. The seat back should support the spine during resting periods when the client is not leaning forward for function. The client with MD usually leans forward and stabilizes on one arm while functionally using the other arm. Trunk supports which provide guidance, but do not limit movement, should be provided.[29] An anterior support for the chest may prevent the client from excessive uncontrolled forward flexion. A chest strap may suffice for this; however, if the client is too strong or tends to lean into the chest strap, a molded chest plate or a block attached to a lap tray may provide more anterior stability.[30] Such stabilization will allow the individual to flex forward for function, while maintaining the ability to relax back into the system for resting.

Therapist's Liability

The therapist issuing equipment to a client must realize that, as a professional recommending the equipment, there may be a liability issue if something goes wrong. Incidents have occurred in which a client was injured due to improper use of equipment (i.e., choking on a positioning vest). The therapist must take care to safeguard against potential legal ramifications. All manufacturer's equipment manuals should be provided to the client and caregiver. Proper care and use of all components should be demonstrated. The therapist is wise to document that this has been done with a signature from the caretaker or client stating that safety and proper use of the equipment was demonstrated. When any modifications are made to a piece of equipment, the therapist must determine whether the warranty on the product was voided. The client should be informed if this is the case. Manufacturers, rehab. equipment companies, and clinicians are beginning to work together to develop increased safety awareness and proper use for the products they issue.

Further Research Is Needed

Clinicians providing seating as an adjunct to therapy need to document the benefits of proper seating. Ideas for new equipment and theoretical implications should be shared to prevent continual reinvention of the wheel. As funding continues to be an issue, the clinician must continue to demonstrate the medical, functional, and vocational benefits of intervention. Doctors, and third party reimbursers should be shown before and after results to further increase their awareness and appreciation for what technology has to offer.

REFERENCES

1. Bergen A, Colangelo C: *Positioning the Client with CNS Deficits*. Valhalla, Valla Publications, 1985.

2. Trefler E: *Seating for Children with Cerebral Palsy – A Resource Manual*. Memphis, University of Tennessee Rehabilitation Engineering Program, 1984.

3. Taylor SJ: Evaluating the client with physical disabilities for wheelchair seating. *Amer. J. Occup Ther*: 41:711-716, 1987.

4. Adler L, Capoccia S, Lee C. O'Brien B: Decision Making Strategies in a Seating Clinic – The Use of Subjective and Objective Data. Memphis, *Proceedings of Third International Seating Symposium: Seating the Disabled*, RESNA, 1987, pp. 91-99.

5. Bergen A: Putting the Puzzle Together Using Commercially Available Technology to Create Therapeutic Seating. Memphis, *Proceedings of Third International Seating Symposium: Seating the Disabled, RESNA*, 1987, pp. 24-36.

6. Bergmann J: Positioning in Life is Everything. Columbus, OH, presentation at Midwest UCP/Resna Conference, October 1987.

7. Trautman D, Flanagan J, Haig K, Cannon S: Therapeutic Concepts and Technical Management of the Upper Trunk and Head in Persons with CP. Mem-

phis, *Proceedings of Third International Seating Symposium: Seating the Disabled*, RESNA, 1987, pp. 101-110.

8. Hart J, Waugh K, Saftler F: *Therapeutic Equipment for the Developmentally Disabled*, Tallahassee, Public Health Department, 1984.

9. Saftler F, Winter J, Waugh K: Use of a Positioning Chair in Conjunction with Proper Seating Principles for a Seating Evaluation. *ICAART88:Choice for All*, Washington, DC, RESNA, 1988, p. 250.

10. Presperin J: Seating and Mobility Evaluation During Rehabilitation, in *Rehab. Management*, April, May 1989, Los Angeles, CA, Curant Communication, Inc.

11. Bergen A: Seating for Function. Presentation at *RESNA '86 Employing Technology*, Minneapolis, MN, 1986.

12. Neen D, Beaucahmp R, Tredwell S: Muscular Dystrophy Challenges for Technology-Seating the Child with Musculoskeletal Weakness. *Proceedings of Third International Seating Symposium: Seating the Disabled*, RESNA, 1987, pp. 139-143.

13. Silverman M: Commercial Options for Positioning the Client with Muscular Dystrophy. *Proceedings of Third International Seating Symposium: Seating the Disabled*, RESNA, 1987, pp. 159-170.

14. Hobson D, Tayor S, Shaw G: The Bead Matrix Insert System-A Four Year Follow-up Clinical Report. *Proceediings of Third International Seating Symposium: Seating the Disabled*, RESNA, 1987, pp. 70-74.

15. Hobson D: *Seating Terminology-Course Materials for Seating Certification Program*, Memphis, UTREP, June 1988.

16. Payette M, Albanese MK, Carlson JM: Custom Seating at Gillette Children's Hospital. *Proceedings of the Eighth Annual Conference on Rehabilitation Technology*, RESNA, 1985, pp. 412-414.

17. Hedman G, Presperin J: Addressing of Positioning Issues of Head Injured Individuals at the Rehabilitation Institute of Chicago. *Proceedings of Third International Seating Symposium: Seating the Disabled*, RESNA, 1987, pp. 111-113.

18. Presperin J: Positioning: An Adjunct to Therapy, in Kovich, Bermann (eds): *Head Injury: A guide to Functional Outcomes in Occupational Therapy*. Rockville, Aspen Publications, 1988, pp. 125-141.

19. Jones CK: The Use of Molded Techniques for Fitting C5-6 Spinal Cord Injured Five or More Years Post Injury. *Proceedings of Third International Seating Symposium: Seating the Disabled*, RESNA, 1987, pp. 189-192.

20. Minkel JL: Positioning for Spinal Cord Injured Patients. *Proceedings of Fifth International Seating Symposium: Seating the Disabled*, RESNA, 1989, pp. 225-229.

21. Zacharkow D: *Posture, Sitting, Standing, Chair Design, and Exercise*. Springfield, Charles C Thomas, 1988, pp. 237-309.

22. Krapfl B: Seating and Positioning Spinal Cord Patients Post Initial Rehabilitation. *Proceedings of Fifth International Seating Symposium: Seating the Disabled*, RESNA, 1989, pp. 229-233.

23. Kanyer B: Designing a Custom Roho. Niles, IL. *Pin Dot News* Vol 1,(5) December/January 1989.

24. Brienza DM, Brubaker CE, Inigo RM: A Fiber Optic Force Sensor for Automated Seating Design. *Proceedings of the 12th Annual Conference*, RESNA, 1989, pp. 232-233.

25. Neth DC, McGovern TF, Reger SI: Computer Aided Measurement of Contoured Body Supports. *Proceedings of the 12th Annual Conference*, RESNA, 1989, pp. 234-235.

26. Chung KC, Sprigle SH, Brienza DM et al.: UVA Custom Contoured Seating System Technical and Clinical Evaluations. *Proceedings of the 12th Annual Conference*, RESNA, 1989, pp. 236-237.

27. Carlson JM, Lutter L, Payette M: Seating and Spine Support for Boys with Duchenne Muscular Dystrophy. *Proceedings of Third International Seating Symposium: Seating the Disabled*, RESNA, 1987, pp. 144-148.

28. Medhat MA: Management of Spinal Defomity in MD. *Proceedings of Third International Seating Symposium: Seating the Disabled*, RESNA, 1987, pp. 144-148.

29. Taylor SJ: The Seating Challenge Niles, IL, *Pin Dot News*, 6-7, June/July 1989.

30. Furumaso J: Seating the Person with Late Stage Duchenne Muscular Dystrophy. *Proceedings of Third International Seating Symposium: Seating the Disabled*, RESNA, 1987, pp. 149-153.

MANUFACTURERS/SUPPLIERS/RESOURCES

The list below is not inclusive; however, catalogs available through the manufacturers may assist in determining solutions. The list was compiled by Hedman and Presperin as part of a presentation for the 4TH Annual Symposium on Advances in Head Injury Rehabilitation, Dallas, TX, March 3, 1989.

Adaptive Engineering Lab Inc., Building 2A, Unit 3, 4403 Russel Road, Lynnwood, WA 98037, (800) 327-6080, (206) 774-7993

BCW, INC., P.O. Box 422, 207 East 9th St.,Cozad, NE 69130, (308) 784-3617

Otto Bock, 3000 Xenium Lane North, Minneapolis Mn 55441, (800) 328-4058

Canadian Posture and Seating Clinic, 15 Howard Place, Box 8158, Kitchener, Ontario, Canada N2K 2B6, (519) 743-8224

Canadian Wheelchair Mfg., 1360 Blundell Road, Mississauga, Ontario, Canada L4Y 1M5, (416) 275-3960

Center for Studies in Aging, Geoff Fernie, Sunnybrook Medical Center, Bayview, Toronto, Ontario, Canada, (416) 480-5858

Cleveland Clinic Foundation, 9500 Euclid Avenue, Cleveland, OH 44106, (216) 444-5857

Consumer Care Products, Inc., P.O. Box 684, 810 North Water Street, Sheboygan, WI 53082, (800) 255-7317, (414) 459-8353

Convaid Products, P.O. Box 2458, Rancho Palos Verdes, CA 90274, (213) 539-6814

Creative Rehabilitative Equipment, 513 NE Schuyler Street, Portland, OR 97212, (800) 547-4611, (503) 281-6747

Danmar Products, 2390 Winewood, Ann Arbor, MI 48103, (313) 761-1990

Dialoguer Product (laptrays), 620 E. Smith Rd W-20, Medina, OH 44256, (216) 722-4000

Dynamic Systems Inc (Foam-In-Place), Rt. 2 Box 1828, Leicester, NC 28748, (704) 683-3523

Enduro by Wheelring, Inc., 199 Forest St., Manchester, CT 06040, (203) 647-8596

Everest and Jennings, 3233 East Mission Oaks Blvd, Camirillo, CA 93010, (805) 987-6911

Falcon, 4404 East 60th Avenue, Commerce City, CO 80022, (303) 287-6808

Fortress Scientific, 61 Miami Street, Buffalo, NY 14204, (800) 387-3611

Freedom Designs, 18165 Napa #8, Northridge, CA 91325, (800) 331-8551, (818) 886-2932

Gunnel, 221 N. Water St, PO Box 1694, Vassar, MI 48768, (517) 823-8557

Invacare, 899 Cleveland Street, Elyria, OH 44036, (216) 329-6000

Jay Medical, 805 Walnut, Boulder, CO 80302, (303) 442-5529

Kaye Products, 1010 East Pettigrew Street, Durham, NC 27701-4299, (919) 683-1051

LaBac, 8955 South Ridgeline Blvd., Highlands Ranch, CO 80126, (303) 762-8720

Luxury Liners
14747 Artesia Blvd. #113, La Mirada, CA 90638, (800) 247-4203, (714) 523-9704, MacLaren/Marshall (strollers), 600 Barclay Blvd., Lincolnshire, IL 60069, (800) 323-1482

Metal Craft Industries, Inc., 399 Burr Oak Ave., Oregon, WI 53575, (608) 835-3232

Meyra, P.O. Box 2361, Matthews, NC 28106, (800) 833-9962, (704) 847-6264

Millers Rental and Sales, 284 East Market Street, Akron, OH 44308, (800) 621-2630, (216) 376-2500

Mobility Plus (Mulholland System), 215 North 12th Street, P.O. Box 391, Santa Paula, CA 93060, (805) 525-7165

Motion Designs (Quickie Wheelchair), 2842 Business Park Avenue, Fresno, CA 93727, (209) 292-2171

Olympic Vac Pac, 4400 Seventh Ave S, Seattle, WA 98108, (800) 426-0353

Orthokinetics, W220 N507 Springfield Rd., P.O. Box 1647, Waukesha, WI 53187, (800) 558-7786, (800) 522-0992 (in Wisconsin)

Peachtree Patient Center, 3123 Presidential Drive, Atlanta, GA 30340, (404) 457-0700

Permobil of America, Inc., 1644 Massachusetts Ave., Lexington, MA 02173, (617) 863-5222

Pin Dot Products, 6001 Gross Point Road, Niles, IL 60048-4027, (800) 451-3553, (312) 774-1700

Poirier, 2930 West Central, Santa Ana, CA 92704, (714) 641-9696

Rehab. Designs, Inc., 1492 Martin Street, Madison, WI 53713, (800) 792-3504, ext. 1234, (608) 255-2200

Rehab. Equipment Systems, 1828 Yale Ave., Seattle, WA, (206) 624-3123

Rifton, Route 213, Rifton, NY 12471, (914) 658-3141

ROHO, 100 Florida Avenue, P.O. 658, Belleville, IL 62222, (618) 277-9150

Safety Rehab, 147 Eady Court, Elyria, OH 44035, (800) 421-3349, (216) 366-5611 (in Ohio)

Scott Orthotic Labs, 5540 Gray Street, Arvada, CA 80002, (800) 821-5795

Scott Therapeutics, 1132 Ringwood Court, San Jose, CA 95131, (408) 433-3863

Southwest Technologies, 2018 Baltimore, Kansas City, MO 64108, (816) 221-2442

Snug Seat, PO Box 1141, 648 B-Matthews-Mint Hall Rd., Matthews, NC 28106, (704) 847-0772

Sun Metal Products, P.O. Box 1508, Warsaw, IN 46580, (219) 267-3281

Summitt Seating Systems, 9231 Laramie, Skokie, IL 60076, (708) 966-2696

Tallahassee Therapeutics, Rt. 7, Box MLC #13, Tallahassee, FL 32308, (904) 877-0488

Theradyne, 21730-T Hanover Avenue, Lakeville, MN 55044, (612) 469-4404

Therafin, 3800 South Union Avenue, Steger, IL 60475, (708) 755-1535

Tumble Forms (Preston), 60 Page Rd., Clifton, NJ 07012, (201) 777-8004

University of Virginia, REC P.O. Box 3368, University Station, Charlottesville, VA 22903, (804) 977-6730

UP-Rite, 3838 N. 19th Avenue, Phoenix, AZ 85015, (602) 263-1129

Varilite Cascade Designs, 400 1st Avenue S, Seattle, WA 98134, (206) 583-0583

XL, 4950 Cohasset Stage Rd., Chico, CA 95926, (800) 356-3554

Chapter 3

In Search of Power
for the Pediatric Client

C. Kerry Jones

There is no describing the laughter of a child that is taking his
first steps. The parents will be clapping loudly during the stumbling
gait and the exuberance can only be matched by one other feat of
human development, and that is the act of birth itself. After those
first steps, the child's world unfolds and the parents become unglued. They are into everything. The acquisition of efficient independent locomotion is the vehicle for exploration and interaction.
The removal of the training wheels and the passing of the car keys
are but extensions of those first steps. Simply put, it's the beginning
of the child's search for power and the development of their ability
to rule over the environment and not be a passive observer.

Unfortunately, some children will never take those first steps, but
they need not be denied the laughter and excitement of independent
mobility. The laughter sounds the same coming from the seat of a
powered mobility base (PMB) as it does from the surface of the
floor.

Once again, the parents have a chance to come unglued. A child
set loose in a powered mobility base offers some pretty interesting
challenges.

Once fingers have pushed a joystick or tiller into the realm of
independence, lives are guaranteed to change. The simple uninter-

C. Kerry Jones is a Rehabilitation Engineer with the Rehabilitation Technology Center of South Bend, IN.

esting world of "Push me, carry me, get me," gives way to the excitement of flat tires, burned out electronics and dead batteries. After the parents stop complaining about banged up door trim and scrapes in the drywall, they usually admit that "power" was one of the best things their child ever received.

This article is not meant to scare off the potential therapist or parent, but to orient them to some of the common decisions and factors involved in acquiring power.

Three basic categories of information are included in this discussion. These are:

- the origins and maintenance of power
- methods of controlling power
- performance characteristics and environmental concerns that affect the selection of power

ORIGINS AND MAINTENANCE OF POWER

So where does power come from? In the case of powered mobility bases, the only source of power is electricity. This electricity is stored in a somewhat primitive device called a battery. Manufacturers of powered mobility bases claim that as much as 70% of all problems with performance can be attributed to batteries. An understanding of these devices and their idiosyncrasies is a priority in maintaining power.

There are three basic types of batteries: gell, sealed lead acid and unsealed lead acid. The most expensive, but most idiot-proof style is the gell cell. This variety costs twice as much as a standard lead acid variety and doesn't provide as much storage or useable life. Advantages are that they can be transported in an airplane and cannot spill. They are the safest to use and are recommended when ventilator equipment is part of the mobility package. Sealed lead acid batteries are similarly designed to prevent acid spilling and reduce the need for maintaining fluid levels. Some reduction in storage capacity and useable life can be attributed to this convenience.

Most individuals are familiar with the unsealed lead acid battery. This style requires that fluid levels be maintained and there is potential for injury or property damage if the acid is spilled. This variety maintains its popularity by being the least expensive and having the capacity to store the most power for its size. No matter which variety of battery is chosen, it must be a deep cycle style commonly used in marine application or recreational vehicles. Standard car batteries will not provide a long service life if used on a powered mobility base.

Batteries for powered mobility bases are sold by "group size." This is a code for the overall size of the battery package and may be listed as a U-1, 22NF, 24 or 27. The larger the battery group size, the more travel a user can expect from a single charge.

The proper charging of the PMB's battery will assure the user that power is available when needed. Batteries used for power storage in a PMB should be charged frequently and not allowed to run all of the way down. This "deep discharge"of the battery shortens its useable life. The batteries' storage level should be "topped off" instead of run "dry." Most battery chargers are now automatic and will shut off when the desired level of charge is reached. Other factors to consider in storing power are:

- Use only distilled water. Plain tap water will cause premature failure because of its mineral content.
- Charge unsealed batteries in a well-ventilated room. Explosive hydrogen gas is produced during charging.
- Do not allow a metal object, such as a wrench, to touch the positive (+) and negative (−) terminals at the same time. This can happen during servicing and the results are dramatic. Large sparks, molten lead, and exploding acid would put a damper on anybody's search for power.
- The type of charger must match the type of battery being charged. Gell cell batteries require a different type than lead acid. Some chargers can be switched to accommodate the two varieties.
- Check the batteries' fluid level every 2-3 weeks and be careful not to overfill. A ring or notch in each of the fluid cells indicates the proper level.
- Clean up spills promptly with plenty of water and baking soda. Do not let baking soda get inside the battery.

So why so much jibberish on such a mundane subject as batteries? First, these devices cause the most headaches, and secondly, without a reliable source of power, the client may become discouraged quickly. Power must exist before it can be controlled.

METHODS OF CONTROLLING POWER

The wheels of power can be controlled in how fast they turn and which direction they rotate. The speed of the rotating wheel can be regulated in a smooth "proportional" manner or through a stepped or switched manner. A simple analogy of a proportional control is the gas pedal in a car. The further the pedal is pushed, the faster the car goes. The speed is infinitely variable from the stop to full speed. A stepped or switched control is the same as a car driven by a teenager. The pedal is either all the way back, "off," or floored, "on." The proportional speed regulation offers a smoother ride and better control of power and is recommended over a switched system. Switched controllers are sometimes necessary due to cost or functional limitations of the client. Switched controllers do not allow infinite selections of speed, but they can offer a smooth rate of acceleration.

Once a child has chosen the direction of movement by activating a switch, then the PMB will slowly accelerate up to a present top speed. This gradual increase in speed decreases the jerkiness in starting and changing directions. The amount of time the base takes to reach the present speed can usually be adjusted to match the client's needs. Manufacturers of powered mobility bases have recently been able to design their electronics so that switched controllers come close to proportional controllers in their operation. The preset speeds are no longer a limiting factor, but free the user to concentrate on directional control.

The types of directional and speed controls used on PMBs can be separated into the following categories (see also Figure 1):

— Tiller/Handsteer
— Joystick
— Multiple Switch
— Single Switch

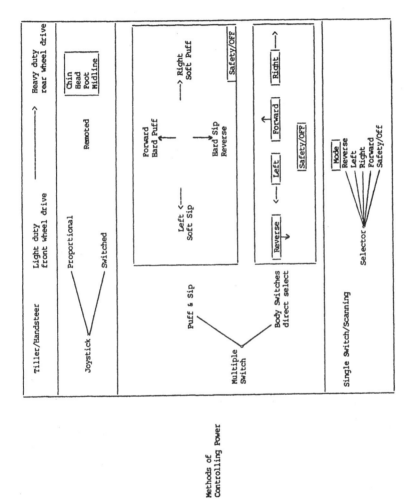

FIGURE 1. Methods of Controlling Power

The diagram and text will expand upon these areas except for the category of single switch. This last method of control utilizes a scanning method for choice of direction. The user must wait until the desired choice is displayed and then activate the controlling switch. A change of direction requires that the sequence be started over. This control should be considered a "last ditch" effort; the first three direct-select methods should be thoroughly explored before trying a single switch method.

Tiller/Handsteer

This classification is commonly called three wheelers and requires that the user turn a tiller or steering device to control direction of the PMB (see Figure 2). Speed and forward/reverse functions are most commonly controlled by switches mounted on the tiller handle. Tiller style PMBs have the advantage of lower cost and much simpler electronics than other types. Because the tiller controls direction, only one drive motor is needed. Three wheelers can be purchased as light duty "mall crawlers" or as heavy duty barnyard rut jumpers (see Figures 3 and 4). There can be a significant difference in needed maneuvering room and care should be taken in choosing the right style. Proportional and switched varieties of three wheelers are available and, in general, the heavier duty models have rear wheel drive. The tiller family has many progeny and companies come and go quickly. Some benefits to three wheelers are not found in other styles of chairs. These include:

—Power elevating seats which can be handy in accessing work surfaces and assisting in transfers.
—Swivel seats which allow work to be performed to the side or rear of the base.
—Ease of disassembly for storage in a motor vehicle.
—The appearance of a scooter, not a wheelchair.
—The possibility of being a narrow width.

Three wheelers may not be appropriate if a lapboard or communication device must be used. The position of the tiller and the necessity for it to move directly in front of the body makes the use of these devices difficult.

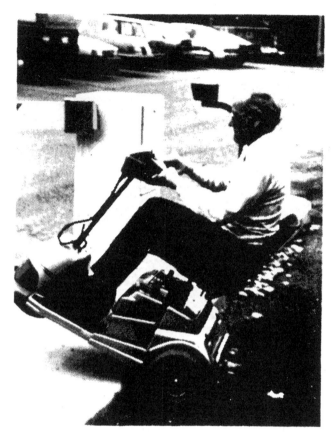

FIGURE 2. Knowing how a base performs allows for a better match between the client and the P.M.B. (Motion Designs ABEC *Sterling*)

Joystick Controllers

This variety of PMB refers to a group of bases that rely upon directional and speed changes being generated through positional changes of a single lever or stick. The act of pushing the stick to a desired position causes movement in that direction. Joystick controllers can be proportionate or switched styles. Not all joystick controllers are created, some styles may be unusable by the client because of how the input signal is processed and then relayed to the

FIGURES 3 and 4. Tiller steering models offer a lower cost alternative and come in a range of styles from the front wheel drive "mall crawlers" to the rear wheel drive "rut jumpers." (Orthokinetics *Bravo and Sierra*)

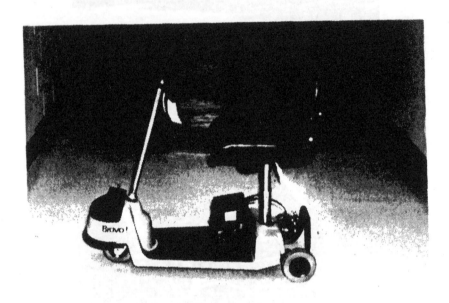

FIGURE 3

motors. The more sophisticated joystick systems allow the electronic signal to be shaped to suit the user's needs. Tremor dampening can be particularly useful for clients that experience extraneous movement while attending to the task of operating the joystick. This feature filters out random signals and allows the client to maintain a purposeful direction of movement. Trained personnel are necessary in order to take advantage of the full spectrum of adjustments. A powered mobility base can be quickly made uncontrollable by a well-intentioned novice of power.

Just because a manufacturer markets and sells a multi-adjustable power controller does not mean that the adjustments will address the client's needs. Trial before purchase is necessary. Examples of areas that can be shaped are: (1) rate of acceleration (how quickly it comes up to speed), (2) braking (how long it takes to stop), (3)

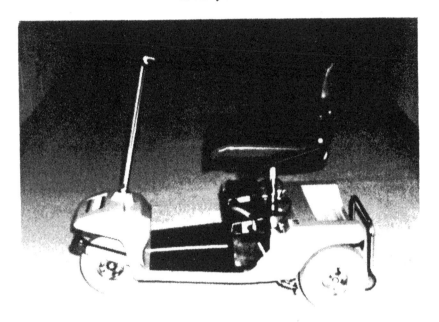

FIGURE 4

turning speed (the rate of acceleration in turns), and (4) sensitivity (how quickly the PMB responds to the input signal). It is easy to see how an overly eager set of fingers armed with an adjusting screwdriver can wreak havoc on what was intended to solve problems, not create them.

Puff and Sip Controls

These controls are designed for clients who can move their jaw, lips, and tongue. An individual with a high spinal cord injury who is ventilator-dependent is an example. The production of air pressure (puff) or vacuum (sip) is achieved through the movement of the jaw and tongue. Secure lip closure is essential for operation of a puff and sip system; otherwise the generated pressure differentials would leak past the input device. Four distinct signals are generated. A hard puff is forward and a hard sip is reverse. A soft sip is left and a soft puff is right. Multiple forward speeds are possible through consecutive hard puffs. This type of system is considered switched and non-proportional, but surprisingly good control over movement can be obtained.

Body Switches

Some clients such as those with severe athetoid cerebral palsy may not be able to control a joystick. Their movement patterns may require that input be generated through gross and haphazard body positions. Individual switches can be placed in the areas that these movements are the most consistent; often the head is chosen. Other sites of input can include, but are not limited to, the hands, arms, legs, and feet. Four switches are normally used that correspond to the four directions. It is recommended that a fifth switch be utilized, if possible, as an on/off site to prevent unwanted movement when the client is at rest. Switches can be built into the headrest, laptray or footboard and should be chosen for their durability as well as ease of activation. A common mistake made by providers of power is the installation of light duty switch connectors. The most popular style is the 1/8" phone jack. These connectors, unless rated for heavy industrial use, will shortly lose their ability to maintain a good contact. Repeated unplugging and stress upon the cord will cause rapid failure. Unwittingly, the family or service personnel will overlook these connectors in diagnosing power control malfunction. Power connectors are the second most common sources of breakdown, next to batteries on a PMB. The flow of power requires a solid connection.

Remoted Joysticks

Frequently, a client could operate a joystick if only it could be positioned in the right spot. Unfortunately, many of the PMB manufacturers are increasing the size of their joystick packages, making alternative placements more difficult. Options do exist that allow for smaller packaging, but these often add to the cost of the base. As joystick packages grow to the size of lunch boxes, therapists are clamoring for midline positioning and chin controls.

When the joystick has been ordered in the right size, or repackaged by a warranty-voiding technician, hardware must be selected to hold it in place. Standard joystick positioning hardware places the control in the prime location for chipping paint off of door trims. Often the only protection device between the $800 joystick and the doorway is the operator's fingers. It is advisable to modify the standard bracketry (if possible) to decrease the vulnerability of the joystick and wear to this potential impact.

Hardware for positioning a chin-controlled joystick is available from aftermarket suppliers, as well as the PMB manufacturer. Consider several suppliers before deciding on the "stock" model. Power must be placed at the optimum point of control.

Foot Operated Joysticks

Few domestic manufacturers market a foot-controlled joystick. Traditionally, good systems have been custom fabricated. The challenge has been to offer the user maximum control without stamping the guts out of the joystick. Devices that use foot positions must shield the joystick from the full force of extensor thrusting, as well as drywall and brick. Foreign manufacturers have paid greater attention to this need area than domestic manufacturers. The source of power has been touched upon and its control briefly explained. How this power is used remains to be explored.

PERFORMANCE CHARACTERISTICS AND ENVIRONMENTAL CONCERNS THAT AFFECT SELECTION OF POWER

Some users of power may want to simply roam the halls of school, picking up lunch and catching the bus home. Other users may want to rip up sections of the soccer field and cruise Mac's for some action. Whatever the intended purpose, models are available to suit the client's particular needs. The difference in types can best be expressed in terms of performance.

How far, how fast, and under what conditions is the base expected to operate? are the primary questions to ask. The therapist may be thinking of the carpet in the library, while the user is planning on competing with the BMX bicycles. Sometimes, the arena of performance cannot be determined because the drastic change from mobility dependence to miles per hour can significantly alter a user's personality.

"How far" is better expressed as range. Range of a PMB is determined by how much power is available (amp hours that can be stored in the battery) and how efficiently the base converts this power into motion. The bigger the battery group size, the more amp hours will be available. Manufacturers usually state range based upon a 160 lb. user riding on a flat surface. Faster speeds consume more energy and will decrease range. How does one determine the needed range for a client? One method would be to outfit a classmate or friend with a pedometer and record the distances traveled. A 50% reserve added onto this number would probably reveal a maximum of 10-12 miles. The reason manufacturers are pushing for a 20 + mile range is that batteries deteriorate and the capacity to store power is lost. Consideration should also be given to a child using the PMB as other children use bicycles. More demands upon range may surface as the weather warms up and school lets out.

"How fast" or speed is the one performance factor that sells more bases than any other. In many cases, how slowly may be a more appropriate question. Some clients need to go as slow as possible in order to maintain safety and confidence. Some bases can go very slow while traveling straight, but can't make a turn from a standstill position. The electronics of the base may allow for slow speed, but sacrifice torque. Torque is the effectiveness of a force in setting a body into rotation. Resistance to rotation may be the threshold of a door or the dreaded ankle-deep, tire-choking shag carpet.

How fast is fast enough? Many adult bases operate with 5-6 miles per hour as a top speed. This is a pretty healthy clip reserved for open hallways and sidewalks. Some manufacturers are touting 8-9 miles per hour with performance plus upgrades. This speed may not sound too fast to the casual observer, but it can be a real thrill! Potholes or caster wobble can be real dangers at this speed.

Imagining the environment in which a powered mobility base will be used actually takes very little effort. Children will try to go wherever they possibly can. No PMB produced can jump across a puddle or climb on top of a swing set, but some models have difficulty crossing a gravel drive or sandy lot. Restrictions upon a child's access to the full spectrum of play can be quickly imposed by purchasing a light duty PMB. Parents may express the fear that if their child receives a powered mobility base, he or she might go into the street and get hit by a car. This is a healthy fear, one that *every* parent shares about their children! A child will get stuck in the mud and may even get lost in a strange neighborhood. Kids are hard on anything that they own. A good dose of safety training is recommended.

Frequent occurrences of trouble may signal the need to reevaluate the appropriateness of a particular base. The author of this article remembers well telling a parent that his child should be more careful when the third sideframe in a year was replaced. The parent point blankly stated that if his son could walk, he'd probably have a broken arm or leg. It wasn't until a heavier duty PMB was issued that broken frames became a thing of the past. The lack of curb cuts in the community and the presence of a rough set of railroad tracks shouldn't determine who a child can have as a friend. On the opposite end of the spectrum, the type of mobility base chosen may be determined by what fits through the bathroom door.

Some of the physical features that influence access on the type of terrain traversable are ground clearance, wheel characteristics and center of gravity. Ground clearance limits the height of an obstacle that can be traveled over. Wheels can differ in diameter, tread style and width. A large diameter knobby tread wide tire may be very effective in taming the back lot, but will destroy the carpet come winter time. A wide large diameter front caster wheel will also decrease turning efficiency. The center of gravity of a powered mobility base is important; if this point is too high, forward or rearward, then the base can be unstable and have a tendency to tip over.

Power can be a heavy burden to carry and how much power is used may be limited by who or what carries this load. As soon as the therapist mentions the possibility of power, the family is already thinking vans and van lifts. It is not always necessary to pile a car loan on top of the 20% insurance co-payment for the PMB. Many schools have buses or vans equipped with lifts and some bases can be quickly disassembled for transport in an auto. The ease of disassembly should be tested by the family member who will be the one most likely to perform the task. A worst case scenario should be envisioned, such as the K-Mart parking lot in the middle of winter. The simple set of pins or latch levers that the salesperson just "popped" into place on the showroom floor will operate slightly differently when packed with snow by a user with a pair of mittens on. Some systems really do work well, but they take practice to be an effective option. The heaviest component that has to be lifted is usually the battery pack. Once the base is disassembled and stored in the vehicle, care should be taken to make sure the components (especially the batteries) are secured in a manner that prevents them from becoming deadly projectiles in case of an accident. A similar issue is the transport in a van of an occupied and fully assembled PMB. A crash-tested tiedown system is mandatory equipment in applications of this nature. Power in motion must be secured.

Add-on power units are popular alternatives to dedicated PMBs (see Figure 5). These add-on units can take advantage of the client's existing manual mobility base for the basic wheeled sub-structure. This combination can allow for continued manual propulsion and makes for a base that is easily disassembled for storage. Sacrifices in performance and noise output are made, but these deficits may be overlooked if cost and portability are the primary issues. The use of pneumatic tires will provide a more positive engagement for friction drive models, but tire pressure should be monitored closely. Tires on friction drive models will have a tendency to wear quickly and traction in snow and slush can be impaired. The manual wheelchair's frame is modified slightly through the addition of mounting bracketry. A battery pack will be hung underneath the seat and drive motors will be mounted behind the back for engagement to the rear wheels. A joystick attachment bracket will be fastened to an armrest (see Figure 6).

Foreign power has become a common option in recent years (see Figure 7). The Canadians have made a significant impact upon available styles, and models from Germany and Sweden are redefining performance and durability standards (see Figures 8 and 9). Some of these bases can come as fully integrated mobility, positioning and environmental control packages. To date, only imported models allow the client to descend to floor level and rise to peer eye height. Prices for imports appear relatively high until a

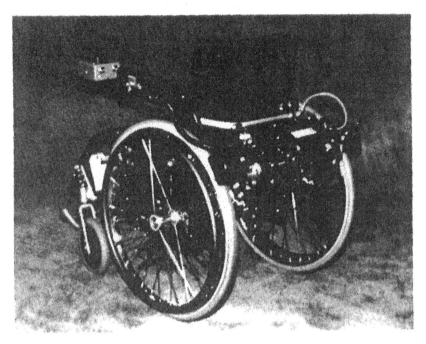

FIGURE 5. Add-on power devices offer portability and lower cost but can sacrifice performance. (Damaco mounted on a Motion Designs *Quickie*)

similar domestic package is compared after all market accessories are added.

Maintaining power is a key issue in deciding what model to choose and from whom to buy. All electromechanical devices will eventually break down. This can be caused by system failure or user abuse. No matter what the reason, repairs should be prompt. Once the dependence upon power has been established, any period of time spent without it can cause emotional and physical stress. Frequent system breakdown coupled with unnecessary lag times for repair can cause a bitter taste for power. The dealer must service what it sells and a strong repair department staffed by trained technicians is more valuable than "special deals" or friendly promises. Study the warranty on the intended purchase and pay attention to the portion covering electronics. Electronic components are fre-

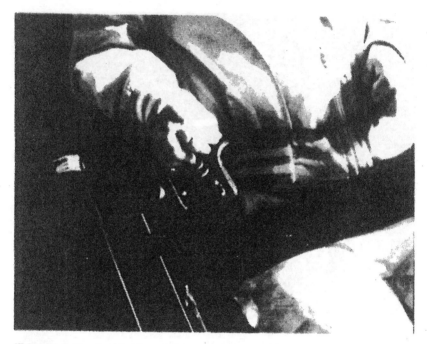

FIGURE 6. Precise placement of a control may require a smaller joystick. (Invacare *Arrow*)

quently given a much shorter warranty period than other components.

PMB manufacturers are beginning to incorporate self-diagnostic electronics. These improvements won't prevent breakdown, but they can assist in the trouble-shooting phase and might prevent the client's power from being returned to the factory when a broken wire was all that was wrong.

Simple care of a base, such as attention to tire pressure, cleaning, lubrication and maintaining battery water level, can significantly enhance the base's life. Change tires before they become unuseable and keep a set of spare inner tubes around in case of a flat (see Figure 10).

A word about aesthetics is in order whenever an individual surrounds himself with power. Style and design must necessarily take the back seat to function, but there is no excuse for flat out ugly.

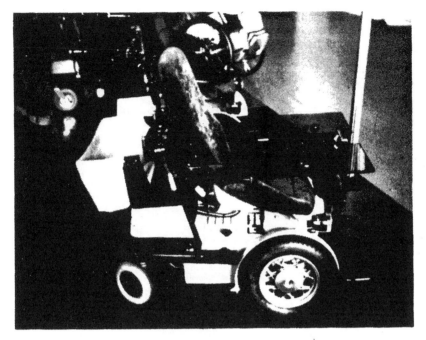

FIGURE 7. Foreign power is becoming more commonplace. (Permobile)

The old chrome styles are giving way to painted steel frames in bright colors, but paint will chip and scratch and these dings will eventually rust. Keep scratches in check with timely applications of touch up paint.

Look for a PMB that allows the *child* to be noticed first. A base that blends into the surroundings is desirable. One factor that influences this ability to blend is sound output. A whining, clanking piece of industrial machinery may be fine on the playground, but just doesn't make it in the library. A base should be quiet enough that a good game of hide and seek is still possible.

So, when is a child ready for power? Barring any severe cognitive or sensory deficits, the concensus is at the age of 24 months. Indications for the need of power when a client already has a manual base include the presence of projection handrims, one arm drive system and the frequent dependence upon others to move any sig-

FIGURES 8 and 9. Heavier duty joystick model P.M.B.'s allow increased access to the client's environment. (Everest & Jennings *Lancer*, Invacare *Rolls Arrow XT*)

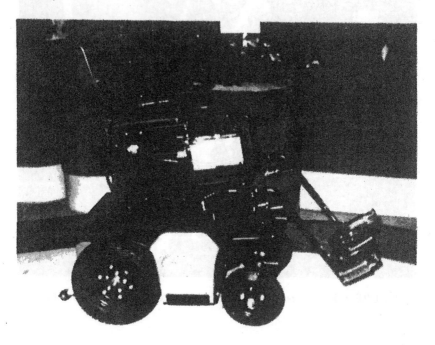

FIGURE 8

nificant distance. Ten feet per minute is not functional mobility and is not conducive to interactive play or getting to lunch on time. It wasn't long ago that powered mobility was reserved until the other kids got their driver's licenses. Attitudes that powered mobility causes laziness and that manual self propulsion should be pursued at all costs remain pervasive and the provider of power may have to deal with such outdated conceptions.

A short disclaimer should be made at the end of this article in that no mention has been made concerning seating and positioning of the user of a PMB. The omission is intentional because a proper discussion of the importance of this area could not be done within the scope of this chapter. Suffice it to say that positioning must

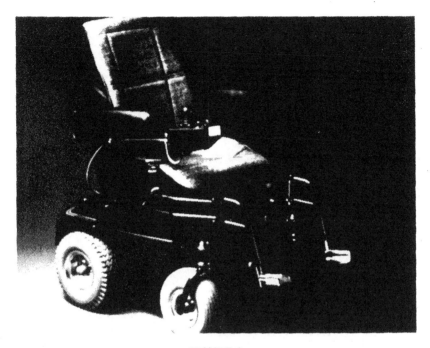

FIGURE 9

precede the issuance of power. True client function and accuracy of control cannot be assessed without such intervention.

   Provision of power to pediatric clients is a pleasure only a few people get to experience. The laughter is addictive and the impact upon the client's level of independence can be dramatic. Power is not to be feared but embraced.

SUGGESTIONS FOR FURTHER READING

RESNA Publications

THIRD INTERNATIONAL SEATING SYMPOSIUM, "Seating The Disabled"

RESNA, Association for the Advancement of Rehabilitation Technology, February 26-28, 1987

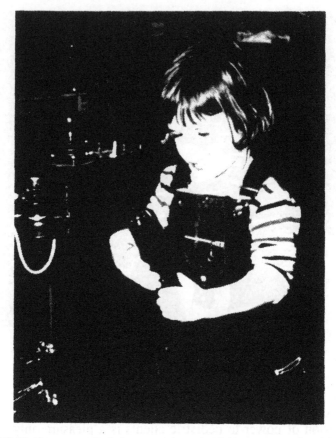

FIGURE 10. Proper service is important in maintaining power, and make sure the technician has been properly trained.

FOURTH INTERNATIONAL SEATING SYMPOSIUM, "Challenges '88 Seating The Disabled", February 18, 19, 20, 1988

FIRST NORTHWEST REGIONAL CONFERENCE
"Childhood Powered Mobility: Developmental, Technical and Clinical Perspectives"

RESNA, An Interdisciplinary Association for the Advancement of Rehabilitation and Assistive Technologies, March 6, 1987

"Wheelchair IV: Report of a Conference on the State-of-the-Art of Powered Wheelchair Mobility", The RESNA Press

RESNA publications are available from:
The RESNA Press, Suite 700, 1101 Connecticut Avenue, N.W., Washington, DC 20036, (202) 857-1199

Articles

Trefler E, Cook H: Powered mobility of children. Proceedings of First International Conference on Rehabilitation Engineering. Toronto, 1980, pp. 113-116.

Butler C, Okamoto GA, McKay TM: Powered mobility for very young disabled children., Dev Med Child Neurol 25: 472-474, 1983.

Butler C, Okamoto GA: Motorized wheelchair driving: Learning patterns of disabled children. Presented at American Academy of Physical Medicine and Rehabilitation, Houston, June 1983.

Paulson K: Psychological aspects of technical aids. Proceedings of Second International Conference on Rehabilitation Engineering Special Sessions, Ottawa, 1984, pp. 282-286.

Verburg G, Snell E, Pilkington M et al.: Effects of powered mobility on young handicapped children and their families. Proceedings of the Second International Conference on Rehabilitation Engineering, Ottawa, 1984, pp. 172-175.

Trefler E: Powered Vehicles for the Very Young: Development Through Mobility. Rx Home Care, February 1986.

POWERED MOBILITY MANUFACTURERS

21st Century Scientific, Inc., 7629 Fulton Avenue, North Hollywood, CA 91605, 818-982-2526
A-BEC Mobility, Inc., 20460 Gramercy Place, Torrance, CA 90501, 213-533-0306
Amigo Mobility International, 6693 Dixie Highway, Bridgeport, MI 48722, 517-777-0910
Damaco, Inc., 20545 Plummer Street, Chatsworth, CA 91311, 818-709-4534
Enabler Wheelchairs, Inc., 310 E. Easy Street, Simi Valley, CA 93065, 805-584-8926
Everest & Jennings, 3233 E. Mission Oaks Blvd., Camarillo, CA 93010, 805-987-6911
Gaymar, Ind., Inc., 10 Centre Drive, Orchard Park, NY 14127, 716-622-2551
Global Research, Box 87, Nobel, Ontario, Canada P0G 1G0
Invacare Corp., 899 Cleveland Street, Elyria, OH 44035, 216-329-6000

Mobility Plus, Inc., P.O. Box 391, Santa Paula, CA 93060, 805-525-7165

Orthofab, 500 Rue Desrochers, Vanier, Quebec, Canada G1M 1C2, 418-681-0667

Permobil of America, Inc., 1644 Massachusetts Avenue, Lexington, MA 02173, 617-863-5222

Rehab Equipment Systems, 1828 Yale Avenue, Seattle, WA 98101, 800-553-9964

Shepherd/Meyra, P.O. Box 2361, Matthews, NC 28106, 704-847-6264

Tash, Inc., 70 Gibson Drive, Unit 12, Markham, Ontario, Canada L3R 4C2, 416-475-2212

Chapter 4

A Developmental Approach
to the Use of Toys for Facilitation
of Environmental Control

M. Beth Langley

Over the last two decades, numerous successes have been reported in teaching young children with disabilities to receive response-contingent feedback with microswitches, electromechanical toys, and other adaptive devices. Experiences with microswitches have, at least temporarily, inhibited development of learned helplessness and facilitated the acquisition of a variety of skills by young and multiply impaired children. Little information, however, is available for using these same microswitches and adapted toys to help children with disabilities to bridge the gap from simple play schemes to environmental control.

CONTINGENCY AWARENESS AND MICROSWITCHES

That children learn to control their world through consistent co-occurrences between their behavior and subsequent environmental results has been well documented. Watson proposed that contingent feedback is necessary for an infant to develop "contingency awareness," a generalized cognitive awareness of the relationship between behaviors and their consequences.[1] Through contingent feedback, young children learn specific responses and develop

M. Beth Langley, MS, works on the Pre-Kindergarten Handicapped Assessment Team for the Pinellas County Schools, Pinellas Park, FL.

awareness and understanding of means-ends relationships.[2] Brinker and Lewis claimed that the generalized expectation that the environment can be controlled is the motivational groundwork for all later learning.[3] Experiences which allow an infant to explore and engage the environment facilitate his differentiation between events he can and cannot control. Initially, infants become aware of their power of control over the environment when caregivers respond quickly, consistently, and reliably to their infants' signals. Children whose experiences and environmental exploration have been limited by severe physical impairments are significantly at risk for failing to develop contingency awareness and, subsequently, for realizing their potential to affect the world around them.

Children with severe motor impairment may convey such aberrant signals that their caregivers misinterpret them and therefore do not respond quickly, consistently, or contingently. The child's signals go unrewarded and caregivers, not sure of how to respond, eventually lower their expectations for competence.[4] Robinson suggested that inability to engage in successful mastery experiences in early childhood arrests the development of self-initiative and achievement motivation, leaving the child with a sense of helplessness and incompetence.[5] Eventually the passivity imposed by severely limiting physical impairment leads to dependency on others, and the child may abandon any efforts to exercise environmental control and succumb to learned helplessness.[6,7] Van Tatenhove pointed out the significant effect of learned helplessness on the development of young, nonverbal physically impaired children.[8] She described this population of children as: (1) communicatively apathetic by two years of age, (2) unaware of how to control their body, objects, or other people, (3) indifferent to their ability to interact effectively and independently, and (4) oblivious to how their unintentional communicative signals are interpreted by others. Douglas and Ryan reported that children whose mobility was restricted during the early developmental years were depressed and apathetic.[9] Robinson stated that learned helplessness is well established by four years of age.[5] Brinker and Lewis cautioned that the inability to understand cause-effect relationships may create secondary disabilities because the child does not have access to normal experiences on which to build more complex behaviors.[4]

Researchers have attempted to circumvent learned helplessness and to foster learning and skill acquisition in severely impaired children through contingency awareness intervention with microswitches and microcomputers. Microswitches have been used successfully with severely impaired children to teach a variety of sensory and motor skills including head and trunk control,[10-14] visual fixation,[15] and kicking, batting, and weightbearing.[2,4,12,16]

One means of counteracting the development of learned helplessness in preschool severely impaired children is through the introduction of play and switch-adapted toys.[2,5,7,8,17-20] Robinson writes that young children can gain a sense of mastery over their environment through activities involving switches, toys, and computers.[5] The theory behind this hypothesis is that once children understand cause-effect relationships they will be motivated to explore their surroundings, which, in turn, will enhance feelings of self-worth and facilitate further initiative. Children who previously would have remained passive participants in learning opportunities can now access learning, recreation, and independent living experiences through micro-processor based toys and technology.[17]

Hanson and Hanline suggested that electromechanical toys offered the following learning advantages:[2]

1. They deliver immediate consequences,
2. They can be constructed easily from toys and commonly available switches, and
3. They can be tailored specifically to the individual child's sensory, cognitive, and motor impairment.

Although it is exciting to consider the potential value of microswitches and adapted toys for physically limited young children, intervention possibilities are overshadowed by concerns that focus on the process of selection and application of adapted toys. On a child level, Behrmann and colleagues and Vanderheiden warn that technology is not a panacea for every severely impaired child.[17,21] Both Annett and Harris and colleagues stressed that the child needs to perceive that the activity is meaningful and related to function in order for the toy to promote continued practice.[11,22]

On the technical level, frustrations that emerge with use of adapted toys in a classroom setting are the time and expense in acquiring and maintaining them. If ready-made adapted toys are purchased commercially, classroom budgets are quickly expended. Durability is a major concern when toys are adapted by the teacher, especially when the toys are used by a number of different staff across several different children. Finding the time to adapt and maintain the toys can also be a problem. If switch toys are incorporated into the curriculum, they must be in working order. Douglas, Reeson, and Ryan stress that the toy must work when the child performs the correct response mode or the child's sense of futility and frustration may be compounded.[20] A critical issue is finding a sufficient variety of toys to adapt that can be accommodated to the individual child's motivational and sensory needs. A large majority of battery-operated toys which can easily be adapted with microswitches emit stimuli that are either too intense for the level of the child's central nervous system functioning, or so boring that their interest appeal is short-lived.[20] Although appropriate, well-managed application of switch-toys can provide pleasurable cause-effect experiences, indiscriminate use of these adapted toys may effect unproductive and maladaptive behaviors and, in some instances, may elicit parasympathetic nervous system responses.[23]

Perhaps the most significant long-term issue relevant to the use of switch-adapted toys is whether acquisition of switch-activating behaviors with toys leads to interactive communication and socialization and to the attainment of some independence in life skill functions via switches and microcomputers. Burkhart,[24] Van Tatenhove,[8] and York and associates[7] cautioned that a switch toy must not be an end in itself. York and colleagues conclude: "Activating a microswitch should not be the goal; rather, it should be a means to attain a goal of increased functional movement or environmental control."[7,p.215] As soon as possible, the child should be introduced to a variety of switch types and consequences as well as to problem-solving and choice-making opportunities via switches. Behrmann and Lahm[18] and Brinker and Lewis[4] emphasize that microswitches should be employed to teach the child to engage and interact with the environment and to select options. Behrmann and Lahm proposed that the child must receive some form of feedback from the environment in order to learn, even if that feedback is from vicarious experiences, and that play experiences engaged in by nonhandicapped children may also be needed and of value to impaired preschoolers.[18] It has been this writer's experience that when children are simultaneously exposed both to play experiences with nonadapted toys as well as with switch-adapted toys, they more efficiently make the transition to using switches for controlling environmental aids than when exposed only to adapted toys. Behrmann and Lahm listed five skills critical to making choices with a scanning mechanism.[18] These five skills can readily be practiced through play with a wide variety of commercially accessible toys. These five skills and an example of their application with a familiar preschool toy are delineated in Table 1.

Children for whom microcomputers and dedicated augmentative communication systems will be a potential reality should practice

Table 1: Using Toys to Teach Choicemaking Behaviors

CHOICE MAKING SKILLS	SEE-N'-SAY
☐ Survey options	drum, ball, duck, etc.
☐ Make decisions	ball
☐ Identify location of scanner pointer	search for dial pointer
☐ Visually track scanner	rotate dial until pointer aimed at ball
☐ Make selection: initiate movement to activate switch	hold handle, pull string

these skills, as they become developmentally ready for the various components, with as many different toys as possible. Examples of toys and play skills important for helping the physically impaired child to learn about, interact with, and control his world are suggested below.

PLAY NEEDS OF PHYSICALLY DISABLED CHILDREN

The world of play and imagination may be limited for the physically impaired child for a variety of reasons. Physical limitations prevent the child from accessing and receiving feedback from toys, and reduced motivational levels may even prohibit the child from trying to engage a toy. Many severely impaired children lack the time to play because of extensive involvement in therapies and other enrichment activities or maybe too sick or too lethargic to participate in play experiences.[25-26] Time must be set aside to allow the child to explore and learn through play, the natural work of children. If a child cannot go to a toy, then toys and other play experiences must be brought to him.

Toys selected for physically impaired children should contain play elements that are developmentally appropriate as well as that stimulate the development of needed physical and sensory skills. This is a tricky proposition for a majority of physically limited children in whom cognitive, sensory, and physical skills rarely match. Toys need to be challenging without being frustrating, and they need to provide the child with immediate and intense pleasure in response to minimal effort. Although play activities are needed that enhance sensory and motor skills,[24,27] even more important are play sequences that encourage a broad variety of imitative and imaginative schemes. It is not unusual to see bright, physically impaired preschoolers' pretend play limited to acting out physical therapy experiences with dolls. Although this form of imaginative play may be somewhat therapeutic, it sadly reflects their narrowed perspective of their world. Riddick offers suggestions for toys for young physically impaired children that encourage development of sensory and physical skills such as head control, eye tracking, fixation, swiping, reaching, grasping, two-handed, and midline play.[27] During the preschool years, she believes that children need to refine eye-pointing skills, develop directed arm and hand movements, and engage in goal-directed play. She cautions that it is important to select toys that have control mechanisms that the child can manipulate or would be able to manipulate with practice. Concerned that if the struggle is too difficult, the child will lose motivation and persistence in manipulating toys, Riddick advises that "it is usually better to help initially and then gradually withdraw your support. Helping does not mean doing the activity for the child; it means *guiding* him in some way so that he learns to do the activity for himself."[27,p.129] Creative materials such as clay, pastry, fingerpaint, and magnetic shapes for fostering self-expression are also recommended by Riddick.[27] Selecting commercially available playthings for physically impaired children is not as difficult a task as it has been in the past. With the introduction of the microchip and other technological innovations, toy interaction is much more accessible for children with limited movement repertoires. Because a number of the most appropriate toys are quite expensive, the caregiver should review the qualities of the toy and compare them with the characteristics of the child(ren) for whom the toy is intended.[28] A brief checklist for guiding the selection and purchase of toys is presented in Figure 1.

Depending on the age of the child, his cognitive level, and his physical abilities, caregivers should consider several qualities of play beneficial to the development of motivation, control, and learning when selecting toys for children with limited movement. Whenever possible, the toy should have the capability of increasing and improving postural and movement potential and control, even if the caregiver must position the toy so as to facilitate a more normal movement consequence.[28] Toys that encourage eye-hand integration are particularly important. If the child is very young or severely involved, toys should match sensory integration needs. Toys which entice weightbearing (the floor piano mats) or provide firm tactile (Playskool's Glo-worm) or proprioceptive (vibration) input (Child Guidance's Big Mouth Singers) help the child integrate a protective touch response. Toys that emit high frequency music or sounds, unintelligible chatter, or sudden or continuous shrill noises may serve to irritate a child rather than to provide pleasure; whereas low

---

Figure 1: Toy Selection Checklist

TOY SELECTION CHECKLIST

☐ Is the toy chronologically age appropriate?

☐ Can the toy be adapted to the child's developmental level?

☐ Can the toy be adapted to the child's response mode?

☐ Does the toy match the child's sensory tolerance level?

☐ Do the toy's qualities match the child's motivational needs?

☐ Will the child have some immediate degree of success with the toy?

☐ Will the toy facilitate new skills in a least two developmental domains?

☐ Is the toy safe and durable?

☐ Does the toy provide experiences different from the child's other toys?

☐ Is the play potential worth its cost?

☐ Will the skills facilitated by the toy be useful in controlling some aspect of the child's environment?

---

frequency, quiet, slow-paced noise toys may help calm and organize a child.

Initial play with toys should provide immediate satisfaction with minimal effort. Electronic toys which produce action and/or sound and visual feedback when the child's hand briefly contacts the toy

(Playfair's Chiggles) or when the child vocalizes (The Right Start Sound Activated Musical Mobile) are now available in large and educationally-oriented toy stores. Mattell's Color Spin and Playskool's Chime Bird are examples of inexpensive and easily-activated toys.

If the child is non-oral, toys that provide language stimulation and that require the child to respond to language are important for setting the tone for communicative interactions. An excellent new set of reactive books, Sound Story™ by Sight N Sound, Inc., contain a strip of pictures which match pictures in the story. When the child comes to a picture in the story and pushes the matching one on the strip, the sound associated with that picture is heard. Opportunities to play with toys which may be accessed and used similarly as a dedicated communication system must be provided prior to assigning a young child an augmentative system. Examples of such toys include the Texas Instrument's Touch and Tell and Touch and Discover, and Video Technology's Talking School Bus. This writer was successful in teaching a child basic scanning and direct selection skills with a broken See N' Say toy by placing pictures of motivational and needed items and activities around the perimeter of the toy and highlighting the point of the selecting device. The child could rotate the selector with a gross swipe of his fist to point to the desired picture. A toy that has served a dual purpose when used with physically impaired children is Play-Doh's Fingles™. The Play-Doh is inserted in a small mold which fits over the child's finger. When closed, the mold forms a puppet onto the child's finger. There are two molds to a set. Turn taking and creative language experiences are fostered by having the puppets talk to each other. An added bonus is the deep pressure applied to the fingers to increase sensory awareness or to facilitate dissociation and stability at the distal joint. A puppet can be applied to a finger on each hand to encourage bilateral activity or shared with a friend to promote social interaction.

Especially helpful are toys that have some type of "tool" the child must employ to interact with the toy such as matching games that light up when the appropriate picture is touched with a wand, or Ideal's Magna-Doodle that makes designs when the child passes a magnetic pencil over the surface. A toy that has thrilled children who rarely have a chance to control or direct anything is a magnetic bingo wand with metal card markers. By holding the wand, the child can sweep it over the markers to pick them up or to transfer them to a large container by scraping the marker on the edge of the container. Competitions can be arranged by providing two sets of wands and markers of different colors. The first child to pick up all the colors matching his wand wins.

The child should have access both to toys which can be activated independently as well as to toys which require some effort to master. If only toys that require adult assistance are accessible, the child may lose interest in trying to play. When the child can experience some degree of success playing independently, "learned helplessness" experiences can be avoided. This may mean that toys need to be purchased on two levels: a cognitively lower level and/or easily physically activated, and a level that will challenge the child's physical and mental abilities.

Toys and games that develop visual perceptual skills and body image are important preschool activities to reinforce. Matching and memory lotto and board games, dominoes, and cards and people puzzles or paperdolls with magnetic clothing are readily available in toy and discount stores. Workbooks requiring responses with a light wand such as Little Questor™ not only reinforce concepts and visual perceptual skills but are self-correcting.

Perhaps most important and least addressed, are representational play and social interaction skills. Because physically impaired children are too often passive observers of life, it is particularly important that they have experiences to "play out" life experiences with representational figures. Playskool's Shuffletown Railroad and Schoolhouse are miniature play sets that have people and cars that are secured in tracks and allow the child to move them from place to place without worrying about dropping or losing them. Playmobile and Fisher-Price Play sets also offer exciting possibilities for imaginative play. Providing the child with a myriad of hats allows him to portray roles of all types of people. The hats are great for encouraging a neck flexion or extension response, depending on the child's needs, for arm and trunk extension (taking off the hat), and for practicing motor skills needed for self-care activities. Battat makes a magnetic stage that allows a child to move the characters by means of a magnetic wand.

Games that require two or more people or that can be shared with other children are critical to include in the physically impaired child's repertoire of toys. Trouble, Hungry Hippos, and Hands Down by Milton Bradley are all interactive games that can be easily accessed with a push or swipe. Buying toys that are enticing to other children is a means of providing the impaired child with a vehicle for social interaction and a topic of conversation. The electric pinball machines and Video Technology's Space Blaster are highly marketable and motivating toys for all children and require minimal physical responses. If a child can only hold the joystick, even through adaptive aids, he becomes an immediate participant in the social realm of Nintendo™.

Toys with keyboards such as typewriters, and Electronic Learning Toys such as Playskool's Alphie and Video Technology's Small Talk are excellent for acquainting a child with scanning, selecting, and motor responses which may be required to activate computers for learning, communication, environmental control, and perhaps, even for mobility. Immediate opportunities to control a variety of events in the environment can be provided through remote-controlled robot toys such as Tomy's Omnibot 2000. Direct computer access to learning and social interaction games can be effected through the Muppet Learning Keys and Touch Window.

Regardless of the type of toy, a primary facet of the child's learning process must entail generalization of the skills fostered by the toy to daily living situations and environmental control. The generalization bridge must be a priority and constructed early so as to further the child's motivational capacity for independence and to avoid static, stereotypic play schemes in which the toy becomes only a means to satisfying immediate sensory or physical needs. If a consistent, organized developmental framework for facilitating play and interaction, such as the Contingency Intervention Curriculum[4] is followed, children will not only be expected to learn from their interactions with the environment but will, in time, and within their unique abilities, develop competence and initiative.

INTERFACING SWITCHES, TOYS, AND CHILDREN

Brinker and Lewis developed a Piagetian-based curricular framework for use in enhancing the young child's awareness of his potential to control the environment.[3-4] The Contingency Intervention Curriculum encompasses the abilities that span the developmental age range from primary circular reactions to simple means-ends behaviors. The six primary hierarchal goals of Brinker and Lewis' curriculum are designed to teach the child to:

1. Explore a variety of behaviors and their contingent results
2. Produce a consistent, reliable contingent response,
3. Use the same response to effect a variety of results,
4. Use a number of consistent behaviors to produce a variety of results,
5. Use consistent behaviors as tools for discovering the types of results they would produce, and
6. Use a variety of different combinations of behaviors to discover different types of results.

Most critical when assessing and assigning a child a switch is matching the child's cognitive level to a compatible form of augmented interactive control.[28] The six goals outlined by Brinker and Lewis above provide a viable format for selecting, adapting, and intervening with toys to facilitate developmental strategies that promote switch behaviors critical to functional environmental control.[3-4] Knowledge of these goals and of the cognitive characteristics inherent in progressive levels of switch behaviors permit the design of an individualized curriculum for teaching a child to make the transition from playing with switches to employing them to access social interaction, improved learning skills, independence, and leisure activities.

Observations of young, severely impaired childrens' behavior with switches suggest that there is a hierarchy of switch difficulty that is developmental in nature and most closely corresponds to levels of imitation outlined by Piaget.[29] Langley proposed a hierarchy of switch acquisition skills based on Piaget's sensorimotor period of development and provided examples of toys at each level that would facilitate the cognitive skill required by each stage of switch behavior.[28] The proposed hierarchy evolved from longitudinal clinical and practical experiences with multiply impaired children and adapted toys, switches, and augmentative communication systems. Three domains of sensorimotor development were targeted as being critical to an understanding of switches as tools of control. Measured by Piagetian-based scales of sensorimotor behavior,[30-31] these domains empirically correlated most highly with switch use. Means-ends behaviors, object schemes, and gestural imitation appear to play a significant role in the child's understanding of a switch as a means to effecting control over the environment, to discerning behaviors appropriate for activating the switch, and for acquiring problem-solving behaviors with a switch. A summary of the development of each of these three domains as they evolve between the approximate ages of four to 24 months (Piagetian sensorimotor stages III through VI) is provided in Table 2. Although there are any number of variations to each stage, the cognitive functions required by each remain the same. Although each stage may represent a discrete set of behaviors, stages may overlap as the child masters one level and progresses to the next. Similar developmental switch behaviors have been suggested by Behrmann and colleagues[19] and Van Tatenhove.[8]

Children first can activate switches whose activating mechanism is not distinguishable spatially or temporally from the reinforcing stimulus. Many times the reinforcer is inherent in the switch itself. Young multiply impaired preschoolers were successful in actively and independently operating the Touch Window to produce visual or auditory feedback but did not understand the relationship between a pressure switch placed directly next to or under a mechanical toy or string of Christmas lights. The rate of responding in this second situation was considerably reduced in comparison to their rate with the Touch Window. Additionally, at this level, a child may engage the reinforcer through random movements which then become systematic as they are consistently rewarded even though the activating mechanism and the reinforcer are spatially separated. The type of sensory stimulus employed at this stage appears to be critical and must be matched to the level of sensory integrative capabilities of the child as well as the nature of the handicapping condition. Children with immature sensory systems prefer auditory, vestibular, and proprioceptive-kinesthetic feedback (deep pressure and vibration) over visual feedback.[32-33]

Table 2: Cognitive Components Underlying Switch Use

PIAGEETIAN STAGE	MEANS-ENDS RELATIONSHIPS	OBJECT SCHEMES	IMITATION
III	Repetitive actions for pleasure; no intended goal	Undifferentiated actions; object & action one & same	Imitates own repertoire of behaviors
IV	Activation for a specific goal; Intended goal	Differentiated actions; Functional use of objects	Modifies own actions; Attempts new behaviors
V	Exploration of different means for achieving goal	Combines objects; Sequential actions; Representational play	Imitates new behaviors he can see himself perform
VI	Foresight in achieving goal; Same means for achieving different goal	Substitutes one object for another; Pretends with absent objects	Imitates new behaviors he cannot see himself perform

At the next stage, children begin to associate their efforts with the consequences when the switch and the consequating toy or stimulus are in direct proximity with each other and to anticipate the consequating action. The child, through trial and error, can differentiate which action to apply depending on the attributes of the stimuli.

Following this Piagetian model, the child is successful at the third stage when the switch and the toy are distanced by a cord or wire of some nature but both are still within the child's visual field. Initially this cause effect understanding is acquired through trial and error and the child may focus on only one aspect of this arrangement, the toy or the switch. The child then learns to shift his gaze between the toy and the switch, and finally, he learns to anticipate the action of the toy when the switch is pressed so that his attention is focused primarily on the consequences of his actions. At this level, the child can discriminate which of two or more activating mechanisms is the one responsible for the desired consequence.

As the child develops the ability to solve problems through reasoning and foresight and can represent his experiences through visual images, he masters the ability to activate various types of switches positioned out of his view for the purpose of directing the movement of a cursor. Two skills are critical to this level of switch behavior: (1) the ability to organize, plan, and respond to the spatial and directional requirements of the switch; and (2) the ability to concentrate on the movement of the cursor, beam, etc. Egan investigated the relationship between cognitive development and use of a switch-operated communication device in eleven normally developing infants.[34] Children functioning below Piagetian stage VI (18-24 months) were unable to use a scanning communication system to make choices between toys.

Van Tatenhove developed systematic strategies for teaching children to actively engage in purposeful switch behaviors.[8] Her assessment/intervention activities direct the teacher/clinician to:

1. Present a toy or device operated through a switch which the child directly contacts.
2. Place both the toy and switch within the child's immediate visual field and ensure that the cord connecting the switch to the toy is also visible.

3. Assist the child in physically accessing the switch, if necessary.
4. Verbally draw the child's attention to the connection between the switch and the toy while demonstrating that action on the switch results in action on the toy.
5. After initial demonstrations, allow the child to attempt to activate the switch and the toy.
6. Allow the child practice time to develop the association between the switch and the toy.

Examples of toys and of comparable environmental objects and activities accessed through the same cognitive functions as their corresponding levels of switches are provided in Table 3. These toys and functional situations are intended not to be inclusive but simply to stimulate ideas of the different levels and qualities of toys that should be available in concert with a similar array of switch-adapted toys and devices when implementing a contingency-based curriculum.

DEVELOPMENTAL SKILLS
AND ENVIRONMENTAL CONTROL

Little data are available that document mental or chronological ages at which children acquire an understanding and use of various types of microswitches and/or adaptive aids. Brinker and Lewis[3] succeeded in teaching 3-6-month-old severely impaired children cause-effect relationships through interactions with computers while Behrmann and Lahm[18] found an 8-month-old to be capable of simple activation of a computer and a 15-month-old to use the computer to scan an array of choices. This level of skill was not substantiated in the study conducted by Egan who reported that scanning skills were not present in children who had not achieved sensorimotor stage VI of cognitive competence.[34] Zazula and Foulds discovered that 11- and 12-month-old children could not control electric wheelchairs but that children as young as 17 months were successful.[35] Everard's[36] infants achieved control over powered mobility at 22 months and Butler's at 23 months.[37] Children as young as 18 months have been observed to be fluent in the use of myoelectric hands[38-39] and Butler reported that two-year-olds have mastered com-

Table 3: Toys as Tools for Teaching Environmental Control Skills

Piagetian Stage	Toy Examples	Switch Examples	Environmental Example
III	Big Mouth Singers Glo-Worm Simon	Buzzer box Mercury switch Light, vibration sound in switch.	Door bell/buzzer Automatic doors Touch-on light
IV	Musical Soft Sounds Bear in Box Color Spin	Pressure switch Roller switch Toy plugged into separate switch but directly next to switch; both visible	Button on automatic hand dryer Button on drinking fountain Electric can opener
V	See N' Say Ambi Tap a Chap Disney Busy Poppin Pals Surprise Box Oscar the Grouch with squeeze bulb	Pull switch Toggle switch Switch & toy visible but separated by a cord or wire, etc. Two switches, each operating a different toy	Light pull cord Elevator button Stereo or VCR button Toaster
VI	Touch and Tell Magna Doodle The Wheel Drive N Play Console	One switch, two activators. Switch locale invisible to child Light wand, eyebrow or cheek switch directs cursor	Remote control TV Remote telephone Vending machines Microwave.

munication systems with speech synthesizers.[37] Douglas, and colleagues did not find that eye switches could be activated by three-year-olds but that a four-year-old could control a four-position joystick held in his mouth.[20] Until there is a larger data base on the cognitive and developmental abilities essential to management of augmentative systems and aids, the existing data and knowledge of child development will serve as necessary guides for facilitating independence and control. York and associates designed a systematic process for integrating microswitches into educational programs.[7] Their design offers a practical framework for teaching switch skills and use of adaptive aids to children in a variety of settings. Among the first of the decisions to be made in such a process is determining whether the use of the intended switch or aid is environmentally valid. In other words, will learning how to use the proposed adaptive toy/augmentative aid be relevant to the child's needs in current or future environments? York and colleagues[7] and Langley[40] have suggested a series of questions to consider when determining whether the targeted intervention is environmentally valid (see Figure 2).

Although systematic, the process is a flexible one and adaptable to individual children's needs. Additionally, it provides for input by all those involved with the child while serving as an integrated plan to encourage communication, consistency, and generalization across all caregivers and settings. The process of York and associates has been modified to be applicable to young children learning to use switch-operated toys and environmental control devices and is presented in Figure 3.[7]

SUMMARY

Current and future technology holds exciting promises for children with severe handicaps. Switch-operated toys and devices have the potential to open a world of discovery and to provide the impetus for self-initiated interaction with the world for children whose physical skills may otherwise lead to passivity, dependency, and a diminished quality of life. Although it is tempting to provide such children immediately with contrived experiences that afford them opportunities to realize their ability to effect change in their envi-

Figure 2: Environmental Control Validity Checklist

☐ Is the objective chronologically age-appropriate?

☐ Is the input graded to the child's ability to tolerate the degree of input delivered?

☐ Does the activity provide preferred sensory/play input in an appropriate manner?

☐ Is the activity enjoyable for the child?

☐ Do caregivers consider the objective important & meaningful?

☐ Will the objective be likely to promote concomitant skills?

☐ Will the activity facilitate postures & movement patterns that will allow greater access to the environment?

☐ Will the objective be useful in current & future home, school, community, or vocational environments?

☐ Will the objective promote socialization with peers?

☐ Will the objective enhance integration into the least restrictive environment?

☐ Will the objective afford more control or greater participation in a variety of settings?

☐ Will the objective facilitate independence?

☐ Will the objective enhance self-confidence & self-concept?

☐ Will the objective expand play skills?

Figure 3: Systematic Process for Integrating Environmental Control Strategies into an Educational Program

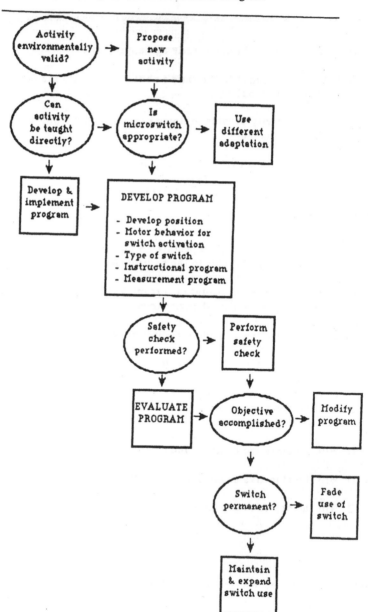

ronment, the importance of play and manipulation of non-adapted toys to the child's overall development cannot be overlooked. Providing the child with play experiences with toys appropriate to his cognitive level will facilitate practice of skills also required by switch mechanisms. A team of professionals including caregivers, therapists, and educators should be involved in the process of designing intervention strategies that are technologically based to ensure success with, functional application, and generalization of environmental control skills and to augment the child's natural development of interactive play behaviors.

REFERENCES

1. Watson JS: The development and generalization of "contingency awareness" in early infancy: Some hypotheses. *Merrill-Palmer Quarterly 12:* 123-135, 1966.

2. Hanson MJ, Hanline MF: An analysis of response-contingent learning experiences for young children. *The Journal of The Association for Persons with Severe Handicaps 10* (1): 31-40, 1985.

3. Brinker R, Lewis M: Making the world work with microcomputers: A learning prosthesis for handicapped infants. *Exceptional Children 49* (2): 163-170, 1982.

4. Brinker R, Lewis M: Contingency intervention in infancy. In Anderson J, Cox J (Eds.), *Curriculum Materials for High Risk and Handicapped Infants.* Chapel Hill, NC, Technical Assistance and Development systems (TADS), 1982, pp. 37-41.

5. Robinson LM: Designing computer intervention for very young handicapped children. *Journal of the Division for Early Childhood 10* (3): 209-215, 1986.

6. Seligman M: *Helplessness: On Depression Development and Death.* San Francisco, WH Freeman 1975.

7. York J, Nietupski J, Hamre-Nietupski S: A decision-making process for using microswitches. *Journal of the Association for Persons with Severe Handicaps 10* (4): 214-223, 1985.

8. Van Tatenhove G: Teaching power through augmentative communication: Guidelines for early intervention. *Journal of Childhood Communication Disorders 10* (2): 185-199, 1987.

9. Douglas J, Ryan M: A preschool severely disabled boy and his powered wheelchair: a case study. *Child: Care, Health, and Development 13* (5): 303-309, 1987.

10. Ball TS, McCrady RE, Hart D: Automated reinforcement of head posture in two cerebral palsied retarded children. *Perceptual Motor Skills 40:* 619-622, 1973.

11. Harris FA, Spelman FA, Hymer JW: Electronic sensory aids as treatment for cerebral palsied children. *Physical Therapy 54:* 354-365, 1974.

12. Horn EM, Warren SF: Facilitating the acquisition of sensorimotor behavior with a microcomputer-mediated teaching system: An experimental analysis. *Journal of Association for Severely Handicapped 12:* 205-215, 1987.

13. Leiper CI, Miller A, Lang J et al.: Sensory feedback for head control in cerebral palsy. *Physical Therapy 61:* 512-518, 1981.

14. Wooldridge CP, Russell G: Head position training with the cerebral palsied child: An application of biofeedback techniques *Archives of Physical Medicine and Rehabilitation 57:* 407-414, 1976.

15. Utley B, Duncan D, Strain P et al.: Effects of contingent and noncontingent vision stimulation on visual fixation in multiply handicapped children. *Journal of the Association for the Severely Handicapped 8* (3): 29-42, 1983.

16. Rugel RP, Mattingly J, Eichenger M, et al: The use of operant conditioning with a physically disabled child. *American Journal of Occupational Therapy 25:* 247-279, 1971.

17. Behrmann M, Jones JK, Wilds ML: Technology intervention for very young children with disabilities. *Infants and young children: An interdisciplinary journal of special care practices 1* (4): 66-77, 1989.

18. Behrmann M, Lahm E: Babies and robots: Technology to assist learning. *Rehabilitation Literature 45* (7-8): 194-201, 1984.

19. Butler C: High tech tots: Technology for mobility, manipulation, communication, and learning in early childhood. *Infants and Young Children: An Interdisciplinary Journal of Special Care Practices 1* (2): 66-73, 1988.

20. Douglas J, Reeson B, Ryan M: Computer microtechnology for a severely disabled preschool child. *Child: Care, Health, and Development 14* (2): 93-104, 1988.

21. Vanderheiden GG: Advanced technology aids for communication, education, and employment. In McDonald ET (Ed.), *Treating Cerebral Palsy: For Clinicians by Clinicians.* Austin TX Pro-Ed, 1987.

22. Annett J: Acquisition of skill. *British Medical Bulletin 27:* 266-271, 1971.

23. Anderson J: Sensory intervention with preterm infants in neonatal intensive care units. *American Journal of Occupational Therapy 40:* 19-26, 1986.

24. Burkhart LJ: *More Homemade Battery Devices for Severely Handicapped Children with Suggested Activities.* College Park, MD, Burkhart LJ, 1982.

25. Gralewicz A: Play deprivation in multihandicapped children. *The American Journal of Occupational Therapy 27* (2): 70-72, 1973.

26. Kielhofner G, Harris R, Bauer D et al.: Play and the chronically ill child. *The American Journal of Occupational Therapy 37* (5): 305-312, 1983.

27. Riddick B: *Toys and Play for the Handicapped Child.* London, Croom Helm, 1982.

28. Langley MB: Selecting, adapting, and applying toys as learning tools for handicapped children. *Topics in Early Childhood Special Education 5* (3): 101-118, 1985.

29. Piaget J: *The Origins of Intelligence in Children.* London, International Universities Press, 1952.

30. Dunst CJ: *A Clinical and Educational Manual for Use with the Uzgiris Hunt Scales of Infant Psychological Development.* Austin, TX, Pro-Ed, 1980.

31. Uzgiris I, Hunt J McV: *Assessment in Infancy: Ordinal Scales of Psychological Development.* Urbana, IL, University of Illinois Press, 1975.

32. Murphy G: Sensory reinforcement in the mentally handicapped and autistic child: A review. *Journal of Autism and Developmental Disorders 12* (3): 265-278, 1982.

33. Schopler E: Visual versus tactual receptor preferences in normal and schizophrenic children. *Journal of Abnormal Psychology 71:* 108-114, 1966.

34. Egan LG: Cognitive development and use of a switch operated communication device for choicemaking. *Augmentative and Alternative Communication Systems,* in press.

35. Zazula JL, Foulds RA: Mobility device for a child with phocomelia. *Archives of Physical Medicine and Rehabilitation 64:* 137-139, 1983.

36. Everard L: The wheelchair toddler. *Contact, (RADAR) 38:* 19-21, 1983.

37. Butler C: Effects of powered mobility on self-initiated behaviors of very young children with locomotor disability. *Developmental Medicine and Child Neurology 28:* 325-332, 1986.

38. Scott RN, Dunfield VA, Richard PD: Myoelectric control system for young children. *Inter-Clinic Information Bulletin 19:*4-5, 1983.

39. Sorbye R: Myoelectric prosthetic fitting in young children. *Clinical Orthopedics 148:*34-40, 1980.

40. Langley MB: The Role of the Neurodevelopmental Teacher in Educational Settings. Lecture presented to Neurodevelopmental Training Course for Teachers, Greenbelt, MD, July 1988.

Chapter 5

Computer Access

Janet Bischof
Glenn Hedman

In the last ten years, the use of computers has greatly expanded in many aspects of our daily life, such as education, work, and leisure. A computer's ability to organize and tabulate information, as well as produce graphics and entertainment, has influenced greatly our lifestyles. In the past few years, use of computers has become increasingly more commonplace in rehabilitation of children and adolescents. Computers can assist one in the achievement of therapeutic goals related to cognitive and perceptual skills, motor function, education, play/leisure, and communication. To provide a disabled child with access to this technology, personalized adaptations frequently require the utilization of hardware and software options to compensate for the child's motoric, perceptual, sensory, or cognitive deficits.

Solutions to accessing technology by the disabled may range from a simple keylatch or software program enabling the one-fingered typist to hold down two or more keys simultaneously, to a voice recognition system which completely replaces keyboard use

Janet Bischof, OTR/L, is Clinical Specialist for the Rehabilitation Institute of Chicago's Alan J. Brown Center for Alternate/Augmentative Communication and Environmental Control, 345 East Superior Street, Chicago, IL 60611-4496.

Glenn Hedman, BSBE, MEME, is currently Coordinator, Assistive Technology Unit, University of Illinois at Chicago, 1640 West Roosevelt, Chicago, IL 60608. Prior to his present position, he served as Director of the Rehabilitation Institute of Chicago's Rehabilitation Engineering Department for five years.

for the client with impaired upper extremity function. Six categories of computer input options are as follows:

1. modifications/adaptations to the standard keyboard
2. alternate keyboard (miniature, enlarged)
3. head-controlled device
4. switches
5. voice recognition
6. eye gaze systems

Determining the optimal solution involves selecting the most efficient yet least restrictive (or different from the standard keyboard) system that facilitates use of the individual's functional movements and abilities. The input method is the manner by which the client enters information into the computer (i.e., the keyboard or a switch). The output method is the type of feedback the client receives from his/her input (i.e., visual information on the display, or auditory feedback). The simple solutions to accessing the computer often insure compatibility of commercially-available software, require less training and cost than a complex solution, and facilitate better carryover by the client's parents and teachers.

Prior to selecting an input/output method and software, an occupational therapist should assess the client's motor, cognitive, and perceptual status to determine the magnitude of deficits in these areas. The client's classroom teacher, speech and language pathologist, and physical therapist should also be a part of the assessment team, whenever possible. The neuropsychologist may administer extensive cognitive and perceptual assessments. Appropriate seating and positioning should be provided prior to the computer access evaluation.

The occupational therapy assessment should address the following areas:

- wheelchair seating and positioning screening
- psychosocial (client/family goals and client motivation)
- cognitive status (attention, orientation, memory, understanding of cause and effect relations, problem solving and sequencing)

• sensory-perceptual status (visual acuity, visual, motor, and tactile perceptual deficits)
• functional motor assessment

upper extremity:
– active range of motion
– coordination
– strength
– muscle tone
– endurance
– reflexes
– hand function

lower extremity:
– active range of motion
– coordination
– muscle tone
– reflexes
– endurance

head/neck:
– active range of motion
– control
– endurance
– trunk
– stability
– movement

• educational/vocational/play/leisure roles

Based on the occupational therapist's assessment, recommendations are made for computer input/output methods and software to assess in a clinical setting. Available options vary in number for each client depending on one's level of function. For example, a client with minimal consistent movements has fewer options available. A comparison of all options is performed following trials of each method or item. The final recommendation is based on those options which meet the client's needs, and maximize speed and accuracy.

Adaptations to the Standard Keyboard

Many computers' **power switches** are located in the back or side of the computer, and thus are inaccessible to one with limited reach. One solution to this problem is to plug the computer, monitor, and printer into a multiplug outlet attached to the front of the computer table. Thus, pushing the rocker switch on the outlet activates all components. Another solution is to plug all components into a power controller unit, which is placed beneath the monitor. The power controller then activates all components with one push button on the front of this unit (see Figure 1). A variety of these devices are available at computer supply stores.

Keyguards can improve accuracy and speed of key selection when one's coordination is impaired. A keyguard is simply a template covering the entire keyboard, attached with a touch fastener called Scotchmate or Velcro. It provides a surface on which the client can stabilize his/her hand and/or hand or head pointer (see

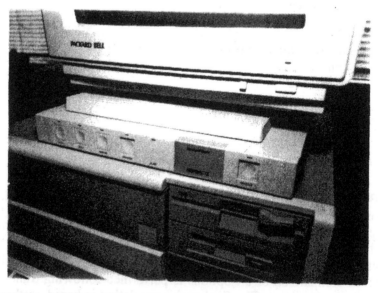

FIGURE 1. Positioned underneath the monitor, the power controller allows computer, printer, and monitor to 'power on' with one master switch, located at the front of the computer system.

Figure 2). Commercially-available keyguards are available for popular computer brands including Apple, IBM, and Epson. They are usually fabricated from acrylic or PVC-acrylic alloy. Examples of these materials can be found using the brand names Plexiglas and Kydex, respectively.

Keylatches are utilized when a client cannot hold two or more keys down simultaneously. The keylatch is attached next to the selected key with Scotchmate or adhesive-backed foam. The keys most frequently requiring keylatches are the shift, control, or a function key. Pushing one end of the keylatch moves the lever over the desired key and maintains the key's activation until the lever is pushed off (see Figure 3). Keylatches are commercially available, and are often already built into a keyguard.

Disk guides facilitate independent insertion of a floppy disk into the disk drive if one must use a pointer or has impaired coordination. The guide provides a flat surface on which the disk is placed and then slid into the open slot of the drive (see Figure 4). Commer-

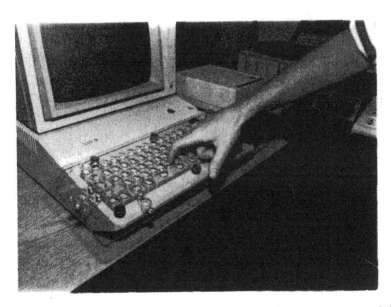

FIGURE 2. This clear keyguard on the Apple IIe may improve accuracy of the user with impaired control.

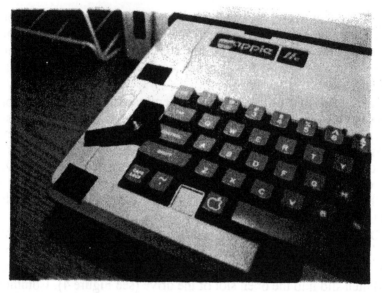

FIGURE 3. The keylatch maintains activation of the control key until it is pushed off and repositioned between the control and shift keys.

cially-available disk guides are easily attached and removed without damaging the surface, thus preserving the computer's warranty.

Keyboard Covers can be used as a beginning computer access method when a program requires only one or two key presses. Each cover consists of two flaps hinged at the cover's top end and attached above the keyboard, resting lightly on top of the keys. A rubber foot is adhered underneath the flap and aligned over the desired key. When the flap is depressed, the rubber foot strikes the key beneath (see Figure 5). The device is a simple approach which allows a person with gross arm movements to make discrete key selections without requiring a switch interface.

Transparent Options to the Standard Keyboards

An alternate access method to the standard keyboard is considered **transparent** when the computer perceives the information as being received from the standard keyboard. Transparent options enable one to utilize software designed for the keyboard. Transparent

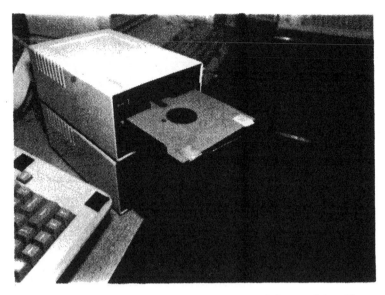

FIGURE 4. The dual disk guides facilitate loading of floppy disks. The metal hook taped to the disk allows clients utilizing a pointer or mouthstick easier handling.

alternate access methods discussed below include enlarged and miniature keyboards, head-controlled systems, voice recognition and eyegaze systems. The two latter systems will be discussed minimally because the complexity and cost limit their use with the pediatric population. They are used primarily for clients with vocational needs. Commercially-available examples of transparent access methods and the respective vendors are listed in the equipment resource list at the end of this chapter. These devices connect to the computer via a keyboard-emulating interface, which transmits information as if it were coming from the standard keyboard and not from a separate device.

The **adaptive firmware card** is a keyboard-emulating interface which connects alternate keyboards or one or two switches to the computer. It also decreases the speed of games controlled by a joystick (see Figure 6). The adaptive firmware card is compatible with some Apple computer models. The **P.C. Serial A.I.D.** is a similiar device which allows alternate keyboards (i.e., enlarged & miniature

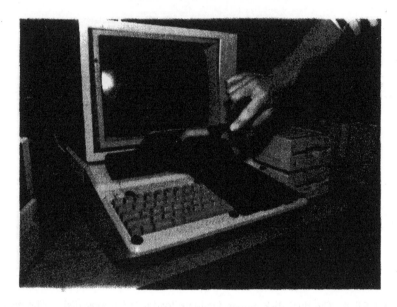

FIGURE 5. The rubber foot underneath the kydex cover is positioned over the desired key, which is then activated by pushing anywhere on the cover.

keyboards) and switches to communicate with an IBM-compatible computer. Both keyboard emulators provide several methods or techniques for single or dual switches including automatic, step, and inverse scanning, single and dual Morse code, as well as assisted keyboard functions for users who input with one finger or a pointer.

Methods of input are classified into three categories: (1) direct selection, (2) scanning, and (3) encoding. **Direct selection** is a method of input where one action by the client indicates one item; for example, typing on the computer keyboard, or pointing to a word. **Automatic scanning** is a method whereby a switch activation causes a cursor to move sequentially through an array of items. A second activation is made when the cursor reaches the desired item or items. **Step scanning** involves continuous switch activations to advance item by item. Although automatic scanning requires fewer switch activations, step scanning is easier to learn for the cognitively-impaired client. **Encoding** is a method utilizing

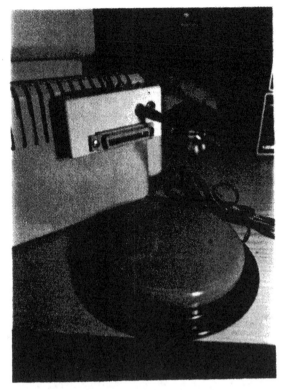

FIGURE 6. The Adaptive Firmware Card provides connections for single and dual switches, and alternate keyboards for the Apple II series computer.

codes to increase the number of selections possible. For example, Morse code can produce all letters and keyboard functions from two switches representing the dot and the dash.

Direct selection is generally the fastest method of input unless the required movement is difficult or fatiguing for the individual. If this is the case, the encoding method would be more efficient for this client. Scanning is the least efficient method because of the waiting time necessary for the cursor to reach the desired selection before a switch activation can be made.

Enlarged keyboards, such as the **Unicorn Expanded Keyboard** or **King Keyboard,** provide an alternative for the client who has good tabletop arm placement but has difficulty when the keys on the standard keyboard are too close together. Both the King Keyboard and the Unicorn Expanded Keyboard require a keyboard-emulating interface. The King Keyboard, compatible with the Apple IIe and many IBM models, has 1.25″ diameter keys which are slightly recessed and act as a keyguard. The Unicorn's key area is 0.8″ square with the keys spaced at 1.25″ center-to-center (see Figure 7). Keyguards are commercially available for 128 keys, or can be custom fabricated from a clear rigid plastic material for larger squares.

Miniature keyboards with keys closely spaced are indicated when a client demonstrates decreased range of motion. The smaller keyboard not only benefits the person who uses one-finger typing and displays decreased range of motion in the arms and/or hands, but may increase one's typing speed when using a mouthstick with full head/neck range of motion. The **Mini Keyboard** is compatible with the Apple IIe, IIGS, and many IBM models. Its keys are arranged

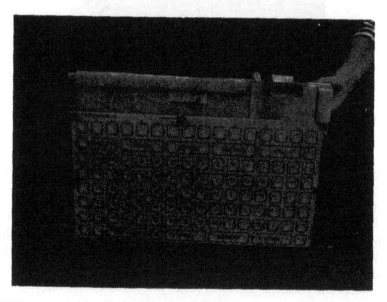

FIGURE 7. An enlarged keyboard, the Unicorn allows for reprogramming of any locations, including dividing it into larger areas, for the user with impaired fine motor control.

with the most frequently used letters clustered in the middle to increase typing speed and endurance (see Figure 8).

Head-controlled input devices are options for clients with good head control but impaired upper extremity function. The input device consists of an indicator worn on the forehead, glasses or a headset, and software which projects the keyboard characters on the screen. The user types one character at a time by guiding the cursor on the screen with head movements and then, either by holding the cursor steady on the character for a set amount of time or activating a switch, selects the character. The predetermined amount of time can be set from one tenth of a second up to two seconds. One commercially-available system, **Freewheel**, provides the user with the option of utilizing a pneumatic switch, whereas the **Personics Headmaster** system requires use of this switch. The Freewheel system also provides a word predictability list which increases speed of input. When the user types the letter "a," a word list appears along with the keyboard image displaying the most commonly used words beginning with "a." If the desired word fails to appear, the user

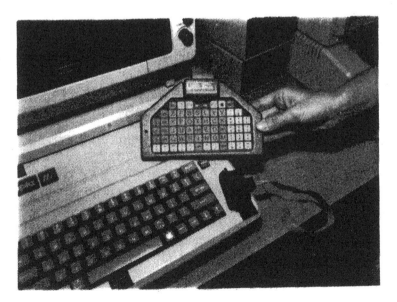

FIGURE 8. The miniature keyboard provides an option for the client with decreased range of motion.

types the second letter "c," and words beginning with "ac" appear. The user can then select the word from the list, which eliminates unnecessary keystrokes. Freewheel is compatible with the MacIntosh and IBM-compatible computers. The Headmaster system works with any MacIntosh system, and performs all mouse functions. Its manufacturer reports that a user could type up to 20 words per minute. The **Computer Entry Terminal (C.E.T.**) is a third head-controlled device which operates by an optical indicator mounted on a headband or by a variety of switch-controlled scanning techniques. It is compatible with the Apple II series and IBM-compatible Systems.

Switches are an alternative for the client unable to access a keyboard or head-controlled direct select system. They can be used with various scanning methods including automatic, step, and inverse, or an encoding method. Switches can operate commercially-available software via a keyboard emulator, such as the adaptive firmware card or P.C. A.I.D., for example. A significant number of switches are commercially available that may fit a client's need. Many cost-saving resources on fabrication of switches also exist. Switches vary in the type of sensory feedback provided (i.e., auditory, tactile, visual, or a combination of these cues); they also vary in the amount of pressure (can vary from zero ounces up to one pound of pressure) and user's body movement required for activation.

The identified feedback stimulus, amount of pressure and movement capabilities of the user provide the basis for the switch recommendation and ultimate selection. Choosing the appropriate switch for a client begins with the occupational therapy assessment and continues through trial training with each appropriate switch.

Some of the most commonly used switches for computer access are the plate, rocker, pneumatic, joystick, tread, and leaf (see Figures 9, 10 & 11). The plate switch is a single switch activated by depressing the plate on one specific edge. The pressure required varies with the manufacturer, usually from 2-7 ounces. It is usually activated by the hand, head, knee, or foot, and provides auditory feedback.

The rocker switch can be either a single or dual switch, activated by depression of either side of the plate. Single rocker switches are

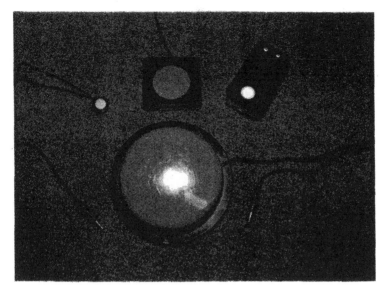

FIGURE 9. Switch options: (left to right) TASH minicup, TASH plate, Don Johnston Developmental Equipment plate, Ablenet Switch 100.

usually activated by the arm, hand, leg, foot or head, whereas the dual rocker switch is most commonly activated by the hand.

The tread switch is a single switch activated by depression of one edge. It provides an auditory click, a spring action sensory feedback, and requires approximately sixteen ounces of pressure to activate. A joystick resembles a toggle and provides a lever which can be activated by the arm, hand, or foot. The pneumatic switch can be a single or dual switch, activated by a sip and/or puff, and is usually mounted on a flexible gooseneck arm.

The leaf switch is a single, thin, flexible switch activated by deflection in either direction. It provides no auditory feedback, but is easily mounted for use with the head, arm, hand, or leg.

The mercury switch is another single switch recommended for training purposes because it is activated by a positional change, such as extending the neck from a flexed position. The mercury switch can be attached onto a visor, barrette, or headband (see Figure 10).

Non-Transparent Keyboards are able to run only software spe-

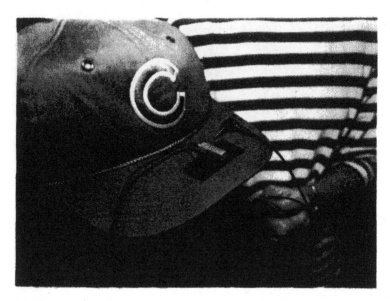

FIGURE 10. The TASH mecury switch can be positioned on a visor to be activated by head/neck extension. The switch would turn off with head/neck flexion.

cifically written for that device. They connect to the back of the computer via the game port where the joystick would normally be connected. As these keyboards have limited software written for them, they are utilized more often in a setting in which multiple clients have access to a device. The limited software negates sole use of this device for clients needing a long-term input system. Examples of non-transparent keyboards include the Koala Pad, Muppet Learning Keys, Power Pad, and the Touch Window.

The **Koala Pad** is a pressure-sensitive sketch pad activated by a finger or stylus and two touch switches. The amount of pressure which needs to be maintained to activate the switch may be difficult for the client with weak upper extremities. The Koala Pad is compatible with the Apple II series computer. **Muppet Learning Keys** is a colorful expanded-membrane keyboard for young children with a combination of letters, colors, and numbers on it. It is also compatible with the Apple II series computer (see Figure 12).

The **Power Pad** is a touch-sensitive 12″ by 12″ keyboard, compatible with the Apple II series, Atari, Commodore, TRS-80, VIC

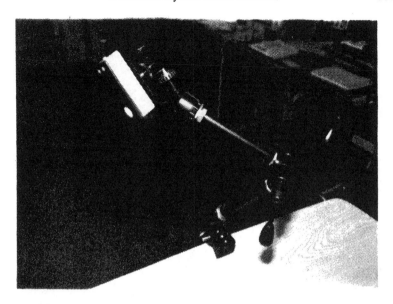

FIGURE 11. The Universal Switch Mounting Kit provides fast and easy respositioning of a switch for evaluation purposes.

20, and IBM PC computers. It includes overlays, a type of coversheet for the pad, that are programmed for many communication and education programs, as well as blank overlays for custom designing. The surface of the Power Pad can be divided into various sized areas, and then that area redefined for a particular program.

The **Touch Window**, when attached to the monitor requires the client to touch the screen with a finger or pointer. If one's reach is limited, the Touch Window can be removed and utilized as a graphics tablet. Software programs commercially available for this device include word processing, spread sheets, recreational and educational programs. The Touch Window may work well for the client with impaired cognitive skills because it entirely negates use of the keyboard.

Voice Recognition is one of the newer approaches to computer access for the disabled, providing computer input by speaking into a microphone. It is utilized in conjunction with the keyboard by the able-bodied population to input multiple key sequences or commands to increase efficiency. For the disabled client with limited or

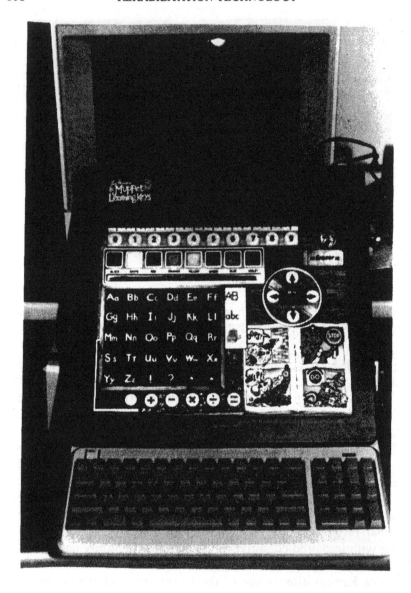

FIGURE 12. Muppett Learning Keys is an alternate enlarged keyboard for the Apple II series for the young child.

no functional use of their upper extremities, all input can be entered through voice recognition. This eliminates the need for any keyboard use.

A training period is necessary to enable the computer to learn the individual's voice pattern, and thus recognize each utterance. The user must speak every word or phrase, as well as the alphabet and numbers, 4-10 times. Untrained words, which include rarely used words, can be entered character by character.

Various microphone styles can be utilized in voice recognition including headset, table or wireless styles. The table microphone may provide total independence for the user unable to position the headset or wireless mike. Commercially-available voice recognition systems vary significantly in capabilities, cost, recognition rate, and size of vocabulary and are compatible with both IBM and Apple II series computers.

Eye Gaze Systems have been developed for the severely disabled non-verbal population unable to efficiently access a communication or computer system with any of the methods described previously. Common diagnoses of this population include quadriplegia, amyotrophic lateral sclerosis, muscular dystrophy, and cerebral palsy.

Computer access is accomplished with the user positioned in front of the monitor in a stable position and maintaining the head relatively still. Systems vary in their tolerance for any head movement. The user makes a selection by gazing at the desired character, symbol, picture, or phrase on the screen for a predetermined length of time. Selections continue to be made by the user visually scanning the screen and periodically stopping to maintain a gaze on the desired item. The computer detects this process via a camera directed at the eye which detects its position by a light reflection from a specific area. This information is then relayed back to the computer.

The few commercially-available systems vary significantly in capability, cost, and allowance for head movement during activation. One system, called the **Eyetyper,** allows no head movement during operation of the system. Another commercially available option, the **Eyegaze Computer System,** allows minimal head movement, although the current cost is prohibitive for many potential users.

Despite these limitations, eyegaze systems can provide communication, control, and increased independence for the severely disabled client who is unable to use more conventional methods of accessing a computer.

AUGMENTATIVE COMMUNICATION SYSTEMS

Computer access can also be accomplished through several types of Augmentative Communication Systems. A keyboard-emulating interface in the form of a cable is necessary for communication between the computer and the Augmentative Communication System to allow use of all commercially-available software. Integrating the Augumentative Communication System and computer offers several advantages including:

1. less equipment, eliminating the need for a second control interface for the computer
2. less costly
3. easier setup as user does not have to reposition Augmentative Communication System to set up a second interface

A disadvantage of a combined system is the inability to access the computer if an Augmentative Communication System breakdown occurs.

Software Options

For children operating the keyboard with one finger, a mouthstick, or a headpointer, software is available which enables the user to depress the CONTROL, SHIFT, or similar keys and have the computer consider the key "held down" until after the next key is hit. The computer then considers the "held" key released. **One Finger** from the **Trace Research and Development Center** is an example of this type of software.

For users who have trouble removing their hand or assistive device quickly enough to prevent the activated key from "repeating," software such as **KeyUp** from **Ability Systems Corporation** is available. This changes the activation from the depression of the key to the *upstroke* of the key. **One Finger** allows the time activating the "repeat" of the key to be adjusted. These software programs which alter the activation of the keys can be turned off when their function is not needed and they operate simultaneously with other programs.

Abbreviation expansion programs increase efficiency of the user operating the keyboard with one finger, a mouthstick, or headpointer, or using another alternative computer access method, such as switches or an enlarged keyboard. The user programs frequently used words, phrases, or even a short document under one or two characters. The stored message is retrieved by selecting only two or three characters. A user's typing speed and endurance can improve significantly with these programs, which also decrease frustration. **Quickey** from the **Trace Research and Development Center** is one example of this type of software. Versions of this type of program are occasionally built into word processing programs.

CONSIDERATIONS FOR CLIENTS WITH COGNITIVE/PERCEPTUAL DEFICITS

When using the computer to remediate cognitive and perceptual deficits, it is recommended that the occupational therapist collaborate with the neuropsychologist and speech and language pathologist to insure the selection of the most appropriate computer programs. An ever-growing library of software that addresses cognitive and perceptual skills is under development, although limited resources are currently available to assist therapists in identifying the component skills that each program actually addresses (see Resource list).

When selecting a program for client use, it is important to consider the method of input required, content of the program, and the complexity of the visual and auditory output. Alternatives to the standard keyboard that require a minimum of cognitive skills are the touch window, light pen, and programmable alternate keyboard, including the Power Pad or Unicorn Keyboard (which also could have pictures vs. letters or words). A few factors to consider when choosing an output method for clients with cognitive/perceptual deficits are as follows:

1. whether pictures or words are required
2. the size of characters or pictures presented
3. whether auditory feedback is required
4. whether a monochrome monitor is required for ease of reading

When choosing a program, several critical factors to examine are:

1. program compatibility with the input method selected
2. the need to allow for slowed responses
3. appropriateness of the vocabulary level
4. quick availability of help commands on each screen
5. amount of visual information presented on the screen at one time

Positioning of the Computer System Components

The actual positions of the input system, whether a keyboard, switch, or head-controlled device, and the output system (usually the monitor) can influence a client's performance as much as the type of system chosen. The client's position while accessing the computer system should be assessed by the occupational therapist and/or physical therapist. Inclusion of the rehabilitation engineer in this process would be beneficial to assess the need for alternate positioning for the client and/or components of the computer system.

Stationary Systems

Obtaining the correct height and angle of the keyboard and monitor, and the proximity of both the keyboard and the disk drives for independent loading of floppy disks, are common difficulties in positioning the equipment for optimal function. Detachable keyboards facilitate ideal positioning for stationary computer systems. The correct angle and height of the keyboard can be obtained with bookrests that provide adjustable angles, or with elevating overbed or standard tables. Obtaining the appropriate distance from the keyboard for the wheelchair user is affected by the height and length of the wheelchair arms, whether the wheelchair is reclined, and the length and angle of the leg/footrests. The adjustable overbed table with a T-shaped bottom can usually be slid in between armrests for the reclined user. Wheelchair desk arms facilitate closeness to the keyboard. Users requiring greater proximal control may need the keyboard positioned on wedged-shaped foam on their laps. U-shaped tables or work stations facilitate the ability to reach all system components from one position, especially for the client dependent with wheelchair propulsion, or the mouthstick user with limited reach.

Commercially-available monitor arm supports which clamp to the table and support the monitor provide a wide range in height adjustment and a narrow range for angle adjustment for good visual contact. These systems require a thorough safety checkout before issuing to a client because some are unable to support the weight of a portable monitor.

PORTABLE MOUNTING SYSTEMS

Wheelchair attachments which provide support for a computer keyboard exist, but the choices are limited. One system, by **Prentke-Romich**, offers a very stable attachment with both height and angle adjustability (see Figures 13a, 13b, & 13c). The system, called the **Wheelchair Mounting Kit,** can be swung out to the side for transfers. Another commercially available option would be the **Quick 'n Easy** system by **Adaptive Communication Systems, Inc.** This system allows easy repositioning of the device by folding it down beside the wheelchair; however, this may increase the width of the wheelchair. In general, gooseneck support is inadequate for support of keyboard weight and the forces involved in the operation of the keyboard.

Attachment of the keyboard to the child's laptray is another option. Figures 14a and 14b show a custom-fabricated, portable folding stand for a keyboard or communication aid. This can be positioned across the lap or on a laptray.

Custom-modification to the child's laptray can achieve an ''inlaid'' position of the computer keyboard, if this is beneficial (see Figure 15a, 15b, & 15c). A clear acrylic sheet can be cut in the shape of the laptray to position over the laptray and computer key-

FIGURES 13a, 13b, and 13c. Prentke-Romich Wheelchair Mounting Kit: (a) Assembly, (b) Receptacle, and (c) Custom-made receptacle for storage of unit behind wheelchair, fabricated by Rehabilitation Institute of Chicago's Rehabilitation Engineering Department.

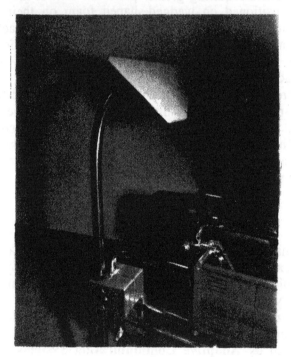

FIGURE 13a

board to protect it when not in use. Clearance between the bottom of the laptray and the client's lap must be present when considering this arrangement.

SUMMARY

Computer use has become a daily living skill for many disabled clients. Therapists must gain the awareness and knowledge of existing technology adequate to meet their client's goals. This goal can be attained by the therapist gaining the expertise personally or by

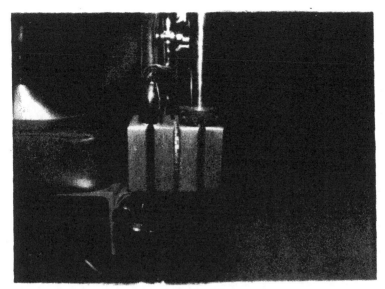

FIGURE 13b

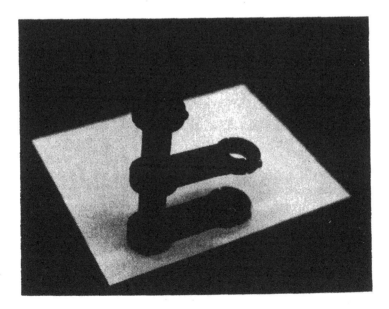

FIGURE 13c

FIGURES 14a and 14b. Folding stand for lap or laptray, fabricated by Rehabilitation Institute of Chicago's Rehabilitation Engineering Department, in folded (a) and upright (b) positions. Shown supporting a communication aid, the design can also be used for supporting a computer keyboard.

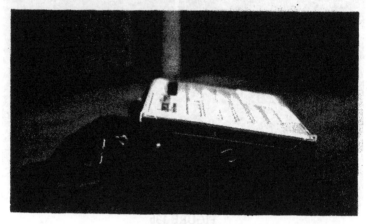

FIGURE 14a

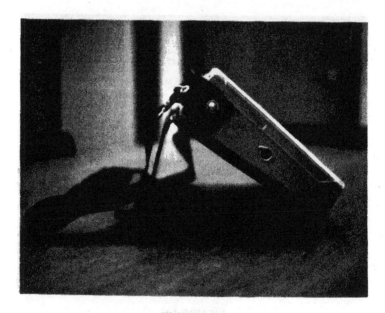

FIGURE 14b

FIGURES 15a, 15b, and 15c. Keyboard inlaid in laptray surface so that better arm support is achieved when operating the device.

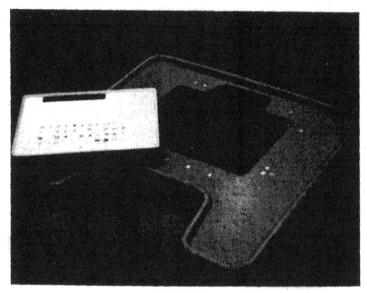

FIGURE 15a

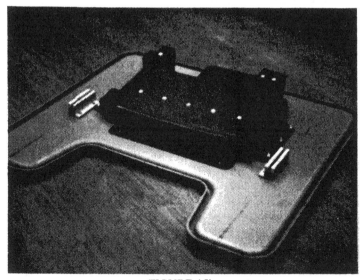

FIGURE 15b

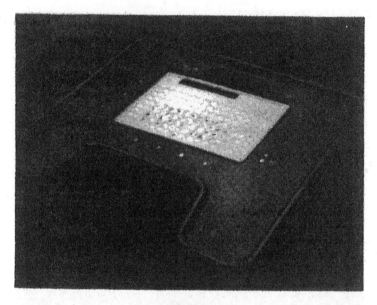

FIGURE 15c

referring the client to a clinician specialized in this fast-growing field of computer technology. The appropriate selection of available technology can have a significant, impact on a client's performance in educational and vocational pursuits.

RESOURCES

AOTA INFORMATION PACKET ON COMPUTERS, AOTA PRODUCTS 11383 Piccard Drive, Rockville, MD 20850
BURKHART, L., *(1984)* USING COMPUTERS AND SPEECH SYNTHESIS TO FACILITATE COMMUNICATIVE INTERACTION WITH YOUNG AND/OR SEVERELY HANDICAPPED CHILDREN, 8503 Rhode Island Avenue, College Park, MD 20740
CLOSING THE GAP, P.O. Box 68, Henderson, MN 56044
COMMITTEE ON PERSONAL COMPUTERS AND THE HANDICAPPED, 2030 W. Irving Park Road, Chicago, IL 60618
IBM NATIONAL SUPPORT CENTER FOR PERSONS WITH DISABILITIES, P.O. Box 2150 (A0651), Atlanta, GA 30055, (800) IBM-2133
MCWILLIAMS, P.A., *(1984)*, PERSONAL COMPUTERS & THE DISABLED, Garden City, NY: Doubleday

OFFICE OF SPECIAL EDUCATION, APPLE COMPUTER, INC., 20525
Marian Avenue, Cupertino, CA 95014, (408) 996-1010

REHAB/EDUCATION TECHNOLOGY/RESOURCEBOOK SERIES:

**COMMUNICATION, CONTROL, AND COMPUTER ACCESS FOR DIS-
ABLED AND ELDERLY INDIVIDUALS,**
TRACE RESEARCH & DEVELOPMENT CENTER, 5-151 Waisman Cen-
ter, 1500 Highland Avenue, University of Wisconsin — Madison, Madison, WI
53705
RESNA, Suite 700, 1101 Connecticut Avenue, N W, Washington, DC 20036,
(202) 857-1199
TECHNICAL AIDS & ASSISTANCE FOR THE DISABLED, 1950 W.
Roosevelt, Chicago, IL 60608, (312) 421-3373
TRACE RESEARCH & DEVELOPMENT CENTER, 5-151 Waisman Cen-
ter, 1500 Highland Avenue, University of Wisconsin — Madison, Madison, WI
53705
WRIGHT, C. & WOMURA, M., *(1984)*, **FROM TOYS TO COMPUTERS:
ACCESS FOR THE PHYSICALLY DISABLED CHILD, SAN JOSE,
CA, ORDER FROM CHRISTINE WRIGHT**, P.O. Box 700242, San Jose,
CA 95170

COMPUTER EQUIPMENT SOURCES

Computer Keyguards, Keylatches, & Disk Guides

COMPUTABILITY CORPORATION, 101 Route 46 East, Pine Brook, NJ
07058, (201) 882-0171
DON JOHNSTON DEVELOPMENTAL EQUIPMENT, P.O. Box 639, 1000
N. Rand Road Building 115, Wauconda, IL 60084, (312) 526-2682
EXTENSIONS FOR INDEPENDENCE, 635-5 N. Twin Oaks Valley Road,
San Marcos, CA 92069, (619) 744-4083
PRENTKE ROMICH COMPANY, 1022 Heyl Road, Wooster, OH 44691,
(216) 262-1984
TASH, INC., 70 Gibson Drive, Unit 12, Markham, Ontario Canada L3R 4C2
(416) 476-2212

Eye Gaze Systems

EYEGAZE COMPUTER SYSTEM, LC TECHNOLOGIES, INC., 4415
Glenn Rose Street, Fairfax, VA 22032, (703) 425-7509
EYETYPER-300, SENTIENT SYSTEMS TECHNOLOGIES, INC., 5001
Baum Blvd., Pittsburgh, PA 15213, (412) 682-0144

Head-Controlled Systems

COMPUTER ENTRY TERMINAL, PRENTKE ROMICH COMPANY, 1022 Heyl Road, Wooster, OH 44691, (216) 262-1984

FREEWHEEL—POINTER SYSTEMS, INC., One Mill Street, Burlington, VT 05401, (800) 658-3260

HEADMASTER, PRENTKE ROMICH COMPANY, 1022 HEYL ROAD, WOOSTER, OH 44691, (216) 262-1984

Keyboard Emulators

ADAPTIVE FIRMWARE CARD—ADAPTIVE PERIPHERALS, INC., 4529 Bagley Avenue—North, Seattle, WA 98103, (206) 633-2610

KEYBOARD-EMULATING INTERFACE FOR APPLE IIE & IBM PC—PRENTKE ROMICH COMPANY, 1022 Heyl Road, Wooster, OH 44691, (216) 262-1984

P.C. SERIAL A.I.D.—DON JOHNSTON DEVELOPMENTAL EQUIP-MENT, P.O. BOX 639, 1000 N. Rand Road, Building 115, Wauconda, IL 60084, (312) 526-2682

Mounting Systems

ADAPTIVE COMMUNICATIONS SYSTEMS, 994 Broadhead Road, Suite 202, Coraopolis, PA 15108, (412) 264-2288

PRENTKE ROMICH COMPANY, 1022 Heyl Road, Wooster, OH 44691, (800) 262-1984

TASH, INC., 70 Gibson Drive, Unit 12, Markham, Ontario, Canada L3R 4C2, (416) 475-2212

Non-Transparent Keyboards

KOALA PAD—KOALA TECHNOLOGIES CORPORATION, 3100 Patrick Henry Drive, Santa Clara, CA 95050

MUPPET BOARD—KOALA TECHNOLOGIES CORPORATION, 3100 Patrick Henry Drive, Santa Clara, CA 95050

POWER PAD—DON JOHNSTON DEVELOPMENTAL EQUIPMENT, P.O. Box 639, 1000 N. Rand Road, Building 115, Wauconda, IL 60084, (312) 526-2682

TOUCH WINDOW—DON JOHNSTON DEVELOPMENTAL EQUIP-MENT, P.O. Box 639, 1000 N. Rand Road, Building 115, Wauconda, IL 60084, (312) 526-2682

Software

DON JOHNSTON DEVELOPMENTAL EQUIPMENT, P.O. Box 639, 1000 N. Rand Road, Building 115, Wauconda, IL 60084, (312) 526-2682
PEAL SOFTWARE, 3200 Wilshire Blvd., Suite 1207, Los Angeles, CA 90010, (213) 451-0997
TRACE RESEARCH & DEVELOPMENT CENTER, QUICKEY, 1 FINGER TYPING PROGRAMS, 5-151 Waisman Center, 1500 Highland Avenue, University of Wisconsin—Madison, Madison, WI 53705

Switches

ABLENET ACCESSIBILITY, INC., 360 Hoover Street, N.E., Minneapolis, MN 55413, 612) 331-5958
DON JOHNSTON DEVELOPMENTAL EQUIPMENT, P.O. Box 639, 1000 N. Rand Road, Building 115, Wauconda, IL 60084, (312) 526-2682
LUMINAND, INC., 8688 Tyler Boulevard, P.O. Box 268, Mentor, OH 44060-0268
PRENTKE ROMICH COMPANY, 1022 Heyl Road, Wooster, OH 44691, (800) 262-1984
TASH, INC., 70 Gibson Drive, Unit 12, Markham, Ontario, Canada L3R 4C2, (416) 475-2212
TOYS FOR SPECIAL CHILDREN (KEYBOARD COVERS), 8 Main Street, Hastings-on-Hudson, Hudson, NY 10706, (914) 478-0858/0960
ZYGO INDUSTRIES, INC., P.O. Box 1008, Portland, OR 97207

Transparent Keyboards

KING KEYBOARD—TASH, INC., 70 Gibson Drive, Unit 12, Markham, Ontario, Canada L3R 4C2, (416) 475-2212
UNICORN KEYBOARD—COMPUTABILITY CORPORATION, 101 Route 46 East, Pine Brook, NJ 07058, (201) 882-0171

Voice Recognition Systems

ARTICULATE SYSTEMS, INC. (MACINTOSH), 99 Erie Street, Cambridge, MA 02139, (800) 443-7077, (617) 661-5994
HY-TEK MANUFACTURING COMPANY, INC. (IBM-COMPATIBLE), 1980 Route 30, Sugar Grove, IL 60554, (708) 466-7664
THE VOICE CONNECTION (IBM-COMPATIBLE), 17835 Skypark Circle, Suite C, Irvine, CA 92714

Chapter 6

Pediatric Prosthetics and Orthotics

John Michael

The aphorism, "The child is not a small adult," accurately summarizes the philosophical basis for orthotic and prosthetic treatment in pediatrics. Although the external appearance of pediatric devices may seem to the casual observer to be simply miniaturized adult designs, often a much different set of unique criteria is involved.

OVERVIEW

The child is a dynamic growing organism, physiologically and psychologically different from the ageing, decelerating processes in the adult.[1] Prosthetic and orthotic devices not only must be technically well designed but also must be appropriate for the age and maturity of the child.[2] A keen appreciation for the normal developmental sequence of human growth forms the cornerstone of effective orthotic and prosthetic care.

Even though the biomechanical principles of corrective pressures are the same for adult and child, the impact on the relatively plastic skeleton of the growing child is markedly different. The use of spinal bracing to retard progression of idiopathic scoliosis provides a good illustration. It has been well documented that low magnitude pressures over an extended period of time can significantly alter the degree of deformity that would otherwise develop in the growing

John Michael, MEd, CPO, is Assistant Clinical Professor and Director of the Department of Prosthetics and Orthotics, at the Duke University Medical Center, Box 3885, Durham, NC 27710.

123

child.³ No other modality (including exercise, electrical stimulation, chiropractic manipulation, and the like) has proven more effective at influencing the natural history of this pathology than orthotic intervention.

As our understanding of the natural history of idiopathic scoliosis has improved, we have been able to target more effectively the population most likely to benefit from this approach. The milder curves (less than 20 degrees or so) are now rarely braced, because progression is unlikely. The severe curves (greater than 50 degrees) are now recognized as surgical candidates, since an orthosis seldom permanently influences curves of this magnitude.⁴

In other words, the "window" for optimum orthotic results has dramatically narrowed over the past ten years. The result of our deeper understanding in this area is that fewer children receive braces for scoliosis, but the majority of those who wear orthoses faithfully avoid the need for surgical correction. In the cost-conscious decade of the 1990s, this more effective targeting of orthotic intervention offers the promise of lowering costs while simultaneously increasing the quality of treatment outcome. Parallel trends in other areas of orthotics and prosthetics are expected to continue and to accelerate.

An additional corollary to the skeletal immaturity of the pediatric client is the need to plan ahead to accommodate the circumferential and longitudinal growth that is inevitable, albeit unpredictable. Provision of soft linings that can be removed is one common strategy to extend the useful lifespan of such custom-made devices. In the case of the child with an upper limb amputation, several concentric "nesting" sockets can be constructed, one inside the other. The innermost socket can be removed as growth dictates, much as the inner segments of a sliced onion can be removed (see Figure 1). Extended footplates and trimlines, removable distal padding, and provision for inserting shims to increase overall length are routinely included in pediatric designs.

By careful use of such strategies, we have rarely found it necessary here at Duke University Medical Center to replace orthotic or prosthetic devices because of growth in school-aged children until at least a year has elapsed. As a general guideline, we recommend that the child return for re-evaluation of the fit and function of the

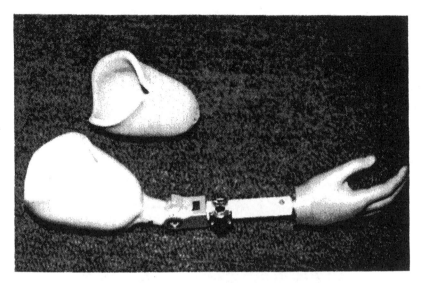

FIGURE 1. Endoskeletal below elbow prosthetic components. Note "nesting" inner socket, which has been removed to illustrate accommodation for growth.

device each time it is necessary to purchase one larger shoe size. In most cases, adjustments for growth continue to be effective until the child has outgrown at least two full shoe sizes.

Growth of the preschool child is much more rapid than that of older children, and in some cases it may prove impossible to maintain proper functioning for a full year. Less sophisticated and less expensive alternatives are generally recommended for this age group, in an effort to reduce the overall cost.

In some centers, the traditional metal and leather orthoses attached externally to shoes, are favored, for this rapidly-growing age group. Provision of a new pair of shoes, or extension of the lateral uprights via growth links readily accommodates increases in the child's size (see Figure 2). Although somewhat controversial, direct formation of splints from low-temperature plastic, fiberglass, or plaster—as advocated by Cusick and associates—is increasingly being explored as an alternative.[5] Because of recurrent problems with durability, such splinting is not recommended for weight-bearing applications on children weighing more than forty-five pounds.

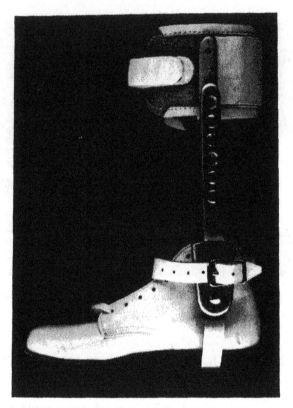

FIGURE 2. Traditional metal and leather orthosis. Attaching new shoes or extending the overlapping uprights readily accommodates growth.

It is of paramount importance to recognize that the orthotic or prosthetic device, no matter how skillfully designed and fitted, is only as effective as the child's mastery of its function. Particularly for the older child with an acquired disability, and for the more complex designs, skillful use training by the therapist is essential for optimum results. Unfortunately, in many areas of the country it is difficult to find therapists with extensive experience or specialized training in orthotic and prosthetic principles. Many pediatric specialists are associated with children's medical centers in larger urban areas; in rural areas, it can be particularly difficult to find specialized assistance locally.

The *Association of Children's Prosthetic-Orthotic Clinics* is one major resource for team members with an interest in this area. Their quarterly *Journal*[6] and Annual Meeting provide an active forum for interchange of ideas and approaches.

The concept of a multidisciplinary Pediatric Clinic Team was promulgated nearly fifty years ago, at the conclusion of World War II.[7] Over the ensuing decades, it has proven to be an effective structure, particularly for the more complex orthotic and prosthetic challenges. At a minimum, such a team is comprised of a physician, a therapist, and a prosthetist-orthotist. Such a "mini-team" can often be assembled even in a smaller town. The resulting interaction among team members almost inevitably enhances both communication and the overall effectiveness of care. Ideally, a complete team might include several physician specialties, social workers, psychologists, and nursing personnel, in addition to the core members.

Regardless of the size of the team, current thinking advocates a shift away from the traditional multidisciplinary focus. By definition, a "multidisciplinary" team contains members from several disciplines; however, each member may continue to view the child from his or her own parochial background. The classic illustration of this dilemma is the aphorism: "A carpenter believes every problem can be fixed with a hammer."

In contrast, an "interdisciplinary" team deliberately develops a perspective that views the child in a wholistic sense and considers the input from each subspecialty as being of equal value. Decisions regarding whether prosthetic fitting or ADL training in one-handed tasks is more appropriate, for example, is based on what seems most promising for that particular child, rather than local custom.

One issue which will become increasingly important over the next decade is the level of qualifications required for team members. In the area of custom-made devices, the contemporary standard for care is practitioner certification by the American Board for Certification in Prosthetics & Orthotics (A.B.C.). Such individuals have met appropriate educational and experiential standards, and have successfully completed comprehensive national examinations having both an academic and a practical component. On-going continuing education is required to maintain certification.

Only those individuals who meet the appropriate standards of the A.B.C. are legally entitled to use the term Certified Orthotist (C.O.), Certified Prosthetist (C.P.), or Certified Prosthetist-Orthotist (C.P.O.). A list of A.B.C.-certified practitioners in a given state can be obtained by writing to: American Board for Certification in Prosthetics & Orthotics, 717 Pendleton Street, Alexandria, VA 22314.

LOWER LIMB PROSTHETICS

The emphasis in lower limb prosthetic design remains largely unchanged over the past two decades. For congenital amputees, the general guideline has been to "fit when ready to stand."[8] For most children, this has been at about twelve months of age.

Infant designs emphasize simplicity, reliability, light weight, and low cost. A knee mechanism is rarely provided because few toddlers can manage a free knee, and most routinely sit with their knees extended. The Solid Ankle Cushion Heel (SACH) foot is used almost exclusively because of its simplicity and reliability (see Figure 3). Suspension is kept as simple as feasible, and most commonly consists of a velcro strap arrangement.

Because the toddler typically has a wide-based bent-knee gait, dynamic alignment differs from that of the adult prosthesis. Because of rapid growth, prosthesis length must be assessed every few months and adjusted as needed. Otherwise, the prosthesis becomes progressively "shorter" as the child grows, and a marked pelvic obliquity with a lurching gait results.

As the child matures, the sophistication of the components is gradually increased in concert with his or her developmental abilities. A manually locked knee is commonly used initially and is later unlocked when the child can master a freely swinging joint.[9] Lighter plastics and metal alloys are gradually making their way into pediatric components, but the major emphasis remains durability. Several hours of weekly play in the sandbox can wreak havoc with complicated mechanisms!

For the school-aged child, continued evolution of more sophisticated prosthetic designs is evident. Endoskeletal devices (covered externally with soft foam material) are appearing more frequently. More responsive foot mechanisms and knee components are gradu-

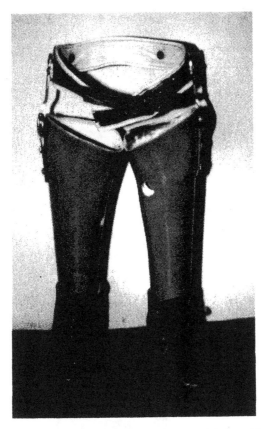

FIGURE 3. Bilateral above knee prostheses. Although fabricated in Cochabamba, Bolivia, these devices illustrate the fundamental principle of toddler prostheses: solid ankle (SACH) feet plus solid knees provide maximum stability and reliability for the small child.

ally added. As adolescence approaches, there is an increased emphasis on cosmetic appearance (see Figure 4).

By the teen years, highly sophisticated prosthetic designs are common. Fluid-controlled hydraulic or pneumatic knees allow varying cadences, and dynamic response feet facilitate active participation in sports and recreation. Specialized designs for competitive sports are worthy of consideration, although many sports are best mastered without a prosthetic device.[10]

FIGURE 4a and b. Endoskeletal knee disarticulation prosthesis. As the child approaches adolescence, the cosmetic appearance of the prosthesis and sophistication of the knee and foot components often becomes increasingly important.

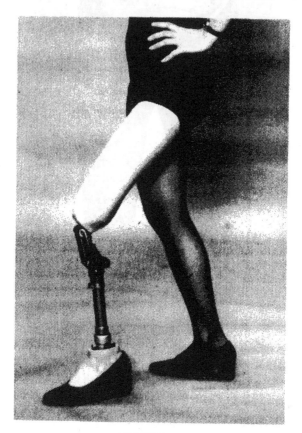

FIGURE 4a

UPPER LIMB PROSTHETICS

Traditionally, the upper limb prosthetic prescription sequences has paralleled that of the lower limb. "Fit when they sit" has been the guideline for early intervention, with most infants initially fitted at six months of age.[8] The emphasis has been on simple, lightweight, passive hands that offer a prop for balance and gross two-

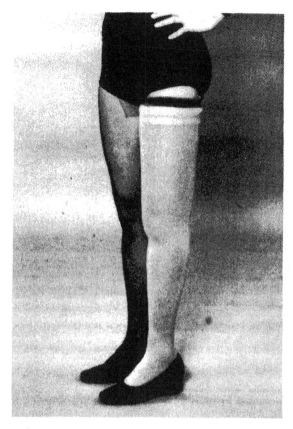

FIGURE 4b

handed grasp (see Figure 5). Particularly for the upper limb amputee, it is important to remember that prosthetic fitting is an *option*.
A substantial percentage of upper limb amputees ultimately choose
not to use a prosthesis, and do quite well functionally.[11]

As in the lower limb, articulated joints have generally been reserved for older children (see Figure 6). Activation of a simple
body-powered terminal device usually begins at about twenty-four
months of age, again individualized according to the child's developmental readiness.[12] In the United States, a mechanical hook has
been the most commonly used terminal device.

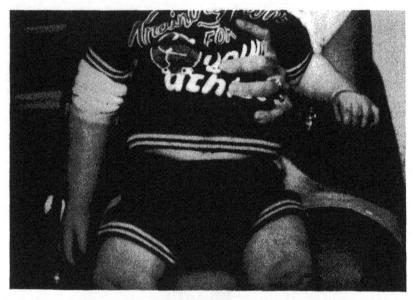

FIGURE 5. Passive below elbow prosthesis for this six month old weighs 3 ounces and provides a prop for sitting. It also helps develop gross two-handed grasping patterns.

At school age, consideration is often given to a more cosmetic device, and a functional hand is sometimes provided. Because the body-powered versions offer very limited pinch force, many centers recommend a trial with an externally powered (electric) device (see Figure 7). Cost, reliability, and weight are the major barriers to externally powered fittings.[13]

By the teen years, as in the lower limb, childrens' upper extremity prosthetic devices gradually become as complex as adult versions. Some centers provide both body-powered and electric prostheses at this age, while others offer interchangeable mechanical hook and hand mechanisms. Although the acceptance rate is higher for electric devices, most amputees ultimately choose one system or the other and use it exclusively. Only occasionally will an individual switch regularly back and forth between two different devices.[14]

In much of the rest of the world, the American preoccupation with functional hooks is viewed with skepticism. Europeans, Cana-

FIGURE 6a and b. Articulated elbow and terminal device permit this young bilateral upper limb amputee to begin self-feeding. The hook is closed by a rubber band, but must be opened by the parent. When the child is developmentally ready, it can be harnessed for active operation.

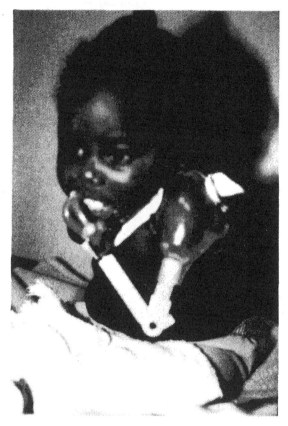

FIGURE 6a

dians, and much of the Hispanic world feel strongly that prosthetic hands are the preferred component. Based on two decades of largely successful use of electric hand prostheses in Canada and overseas, even for very young children, there is a growing movement in American circles to provide sophisticated devices at an early age.

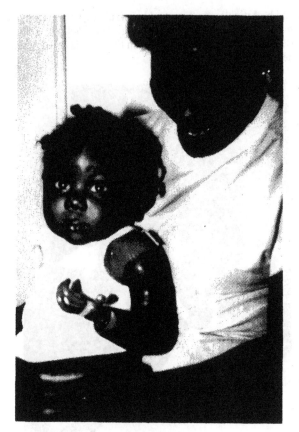

FIGURE 6b

Although an incendiary statement such as "It is criminal to fit anyone with a hook,"[15] adds little to our understanding in this area, it does reflect the sentiments of many parents and much of the world. Most fitting of electric prostheses for infants in the U.S. is performed at selected medical centers, supported by an experienced team of prosthetists and therapists. The results are being watched closely by other clinicians, to see whether these children seem to have an advantage over their peers who are fitted with electric devices at school age or later.

One additional area of growing interest in upper limb prosthetics

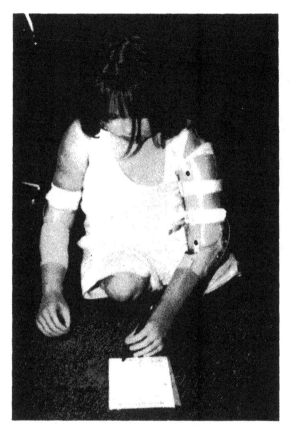

FIGURE 7. This first-grader with four acquired amputations is using hybrid prostheses. The below elbow limb has a mechanical hand. The elbow disarticulation limb has a mechanical elbow with a switch-controlled elctric hand.

is the provision of voluntary closing terminal devices, rather than the more common voluntary opening ones (see Figure 8). The leading proponent of this approach is Bob Radocy, a recreational therapist and below-elbow amputee. He has produced a number of terminal devices that require muscle activity to maintain a grip, including designs for very young children, and argues that the stronger grasp makes the devices more functionally useful.[16] Particularly for unilateral below-elbow clients, these devices are gaining increasing clinical acceptance.

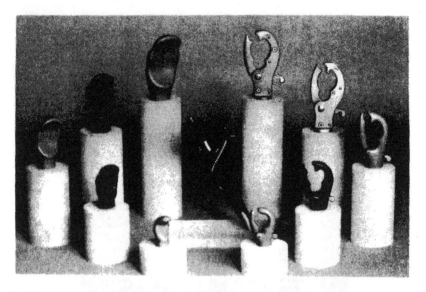

FIGURE 8. These voluntary-closing terminal devices have been successfully used by pediatric amputees, particularly for unilateral below elbow applications. Note also the flexible mitts for sports such as basketball and the attachment for snow ski poles. [Courtesy of TRS, Inc.]

UPPER LIMB ORTHOTICS

Most pediatric upper limb orthoses are interim devices with a practical lifespan measured in weeks. The majority are provided by occupational therapists, generally from low-temperature plastics, and perform quite satisfactorily.

The designs provided by the certified orthotist are primarily appropriate for long-term definitive use, which is uncommon in this population. On occasion, the corrective forces involved will make low-temperature plastics unsuitable. When strong deforming forces are present, such as in radial club hands or elbow contractures, the high-temperature designs of the orthotist may be necessary.

When reconstructive surgery is not possible, severely malformed upper limbs may be ablated and prosthetic fitting offered. In the majority of cases, however, the sensation and range of motion offered by even bizarrely shaped residual limbs may be superior to any orthotic or prosthetic design. Comprehensive therapy to foster ADL skills is then the preferred treatment.

LOWER LIMB ORTHOTICS

Two major trends are emerging in the realm of lower limb orthotics. The first is the incorporation of neurophysiological principles, along with traditional biomechanical control principles, in definitive orthotic designs.[17]

Many differing and sometimes conflicting approaches to the inhibition of spasticity are currently advocated by various podiatrists, physicians, therapists, and orthotists. At the present time, a period of active exploration of various alternatives is underway, but it is premature to speculate as to which views will become the dominant trends.

General agreement seems to exist on three fundamental principles:

1. Avoid stimulating undesirable primitive responses,
2. Inhibit the above, whenever feasible, and
3. Facilitate antagonist musculature, if possible.

One of the keys to reducing spastic tone seems to be meticulous alignment of the hindfoot in a neutral position. Although explanations may vary, most techniques can be summarized as involving careful attention to basic orthotic biomechanical principles.

Many casting techniques are being advocated, each with their proponents. Our approach at Duke University has been an interdisciplinary one. Inhibitive pediatric AFOs [Ankle-Foot Orthoses] begin with footplates fashioned by the physical therapist with neurodevelopmental treatment (NDT) training. These are incorporated into the plaster negative impression by the orthotist, with the therapist assisting during the casting in difficult cases. Positive model modification, fabrication, and fitting are the orthotist's responsibility.

Inhibitive AFOs are never provided in isolation, but only as an adjunct to ongoing therapy with an NDT-Certified physical therapist (see Figure 9). Follow-up and adjustments are performed

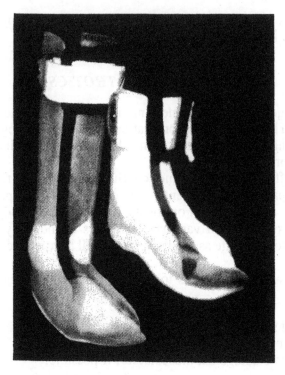

FIGURE 9. Examples of inhibitive AFO's combining the knowledge and skills of the orthotist and therapist. Extended trimlines plus very flexible margins wrap intimately around the leg to enhance control.

jointly by the C.O. and physical therapist, as the child's needs dictate.

In marginal cases, a trial with plaster boots or fiberglass temporary splints is undertaken, prior to definitive orthotic design. As was mentioned earlier, preschool children (less than five years old) generally receive low-temperature splints, because they are outgrown in a matter of months. By the time recurrent breakage becomes a problem, the growth rate has slowed somewhat and the child is ready for more definitive high-temperature designs, provided jointly by the therapist-orthotist team.

The second emerging trend in lower limb orthotics is a renewed focus on articulated designs.[18] Two decades ago, the metal brace with ankle joint was ubiquitous. As thermoplastic designs gradually displaced the heavier metal systems, there was a corresponding shift to solid ankle designs due, in part, to their inherently light weight and reliability.

The availability of several components permitting articulation of plastic braces at the anatomical ankle has opened up new possibilities in orthotic management (see Figure 10). Although durability and efficacy have yet to be thoroughly documented, a variety of free motion and limited motion designs are now being fitted. In

FIGURE 10a and b. Example of an articulated AFO to prevent plantar flexion beyond neurtal while allowing dorsiflexion. Note adjustable elastic strap to resist tibial collapse and lateral posting to improve varus control.

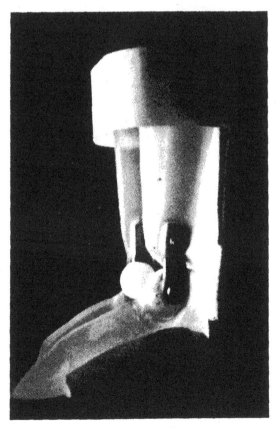

FIGURE 10a

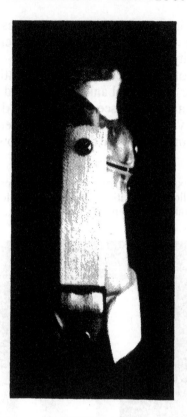

FIGURE 10b

general, children seem to prefer the additional freedom these orthoses provide.

It is quite possible to combine both trends and create an articulated AFO with an inhibitive footplate. Although originally proposed for adult clients post-CVA, this design also has merit in pediatrics.

Specific indications and contraindications for each variation remain under discussion. In general, the more severe the spasticity or pathology, the more likely a rigid device will be required for adequate control. In some cases, the tone will diminish sufficiently after a year or so of rigid brace use that an articulated design can be attempted.

A general trend in lower limb orthotics is to avoid KAFOs [Knee-Ankle-Foot Orthoses] and more complicated devices unless absolutely necessary (see Figure 11). Nevertheless, development of the Reciprocating Gait Orthosis (RGO) by Louisiana State University has significantly increased the mobility of children whose disability requires the use of HKAFOs [Hip-Knee-Ankle-Foot Orthoses] (see Figure 12). Several studies have suggested that the reciprocating foot-over-foot gait the RGO permits requires less energy expendi-

FIGURE 11a and b. All plastic KAFO weighs five ounces yet provides sufficient genu varum control for this three year old.

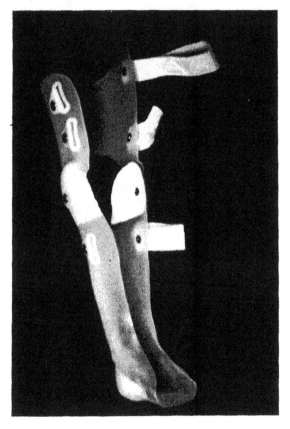

FIGURE 11a

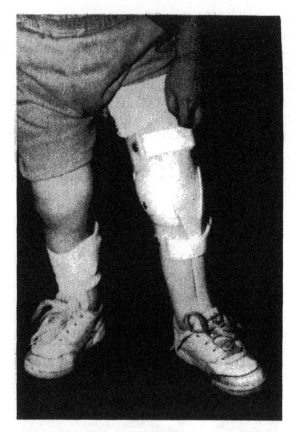

FIGURE 11b

ture than a swing-to or swing-through gait — even though the latter may be faster.[19] Presumably the reciprocal gait is more efficient because the center of gravity is displaced side-to-side but never completely elevated by the arms as is the case in a swinging gait.

SPINAL ORTHOTICS

More precise indications for orthotic intervention in idiopathic scoliosis have already been discussed. A steady trend toward lighter, more flexible, and more comfortable plastics in spinal or-

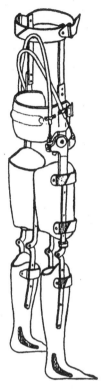

FIGURE 12. Reciprocal Gait Orthosis (RGO) allows many severely involved children to develop a step-over-step gait, which has been shown to decrease the effort necessary to ambulate. This device also permits a swing-through gait, which is more tiring but faster. [Courtesy of Durr-Fillauer Medical, Inc.]

thosis design is also apparent. More effective surgical stabilization of the spine with new instrumentation has reduced the necessity for post-operative bracing. In general, spinal orthoses are indicated for children only as an adjunct during the healing phase following surgery or for non-operative conditions. The orthosis can also be used to defer surgical intervention until the child is older. Effective bracing of the infant and toddler, however, is a very difficult challenge (see Figure 13).

Many prosthetists and orthotists are developing an interest and ability in the area of custom seating.[20] Again, an interdisciplinary

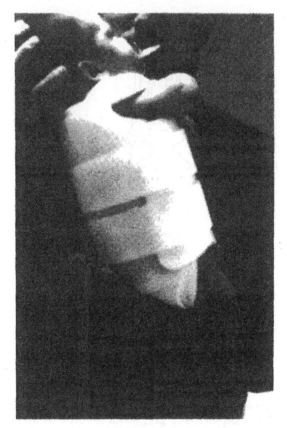

FIGURE 13. Custom-made bivalved body jacket stabilized this infant's collapsing spine until surgical correction was feasible.

team is the preferred approach, ideally including both an occupational and a physical therapist, along with the physician and certified orthotist. Larger centers may enjoy the availability of a rehabilitation engineer as well as technical support staff to carry out the fabrication.

As in any area of custom services, the key is to individualize the seating system for each client's needs. Relatively simple problems lend themselves to straightforward solutions, carved from various foams or assembled from prefabricated components. Very rigid deformities seem to do best with Foam-In-Place (FIP) techniques, which accurately capture the three-dimensional contours of their fixed posture. Complex but partially correctable deformities, particularly if complicated by tone disturbances, may require custom-molded devices based on a seating simulation evaluation. The Contour-U system is one effective approach that uses these principles.

SUMMARY

The fundamental tenet of orthotic or prosthetic design for pediatric clients is to individualize the device, taking into account both the needs and developmental readiness of the child. The general emphasis is on simplicity, reliability, and light weight—particularly for the smaller child. The best device is the least device necessary to provide the desired result.

Advances in the sophistication of componentry and design have begun to reach pediatric practice, particularly in the area of Reciprocating Gait Orthoses and electrically-powered prosthetic hands. A renewed emphasis on articulated designs, coupled with an emerging appreciation for neurophysiological principles, has resulted in more effective bracing of the youngster.

As our understanding grows, we can target our orthotic and prosthetic interventions to be increasingly effective. A multidisciplinary team, with an interdisciplinary focus, maximizes the effectiveness of the devices provided.

A good concluding aphorism would be: "The prosthetist-orthotist designs it; the therapist explains it; but it is the child who makes it work!" Fortunately, most pediatric clients are eager learners, and the majority find that orthotic and prosthetic devices can make a significant contribution to their independence and quality of life.

REFERENCES

1. *American Academy of Orthopedic Surgeons Atlas of Limb Prosthetics*, St. Louis, MO, CV Mosby Company, 1981, pp. 494-5.

2. American Academy of Orthopedic Surgeons *Atlas of Limb Prosthetics*. St. Louis, MO, CV Mosby Company, 1981, p. 499.

3. Blount WP, Moe JH: *The Milwaukee Brace*, Baltimore, MD, Williams and Wilkins, 1973, p. 17.

4. Winter RB, Moe JH: Orthotics for spinal deformity. *Clinical Orthopedics and Related Research* 102: 76-77, 1974.

5. Cusick BD: Splints and casts: Managing foot deformity in children with neuromotor disorders. *Phys Ther* 68: 1903-1912, 1988.

6. *Journal of the Association of Childrens' Prosthetic-Orthotic Clinics*, 317 East 34th Street, 10th Floor, New York, NY 10016.

7. American Academy of Orthopedic Surgeons *Atlas of Limb Prosthetics*. St. Louis, MO, CV Mosby Company, 1981, p. 493.

8. *The Juvenile Amputee*. Chicago, IL, Northwestern University Prosthetic-Orthotic Center, 1976.

9. Sanders GT: *Lower Limb Amputations: A Guide to Rehabilitation*, Philadelphia, PA, FA Davis Company, 1986, p. 534.

10. Michael JW: New developments in prosthetic feet for sports and recreation. *Palaestra* 5(2): 35, 1989.

11. Melendez D, LeBlanc M: Survey of arm amputees not wearing prostheses: Implications for research and service. *Journal of the Association of Childrens' Prosthetic-Orthotic Clinics* 23(3): 67, 1988.

12. American Academy of Orthopedic Surgeons *Atlas of Limb Prosthetics*. St. Louis, MO, CV Mosby Company, 1981, p. 599.

13. Michael JW: Powered upper limb components and controls: Current concepts. *Clinical Prosthetics & Orthotics* 10(2): 74, 1986.

14. DeBear P: Functional use of myoelectric and cable-driven protheses. *Journal of the Association of Childrens' Prosthetic-Orthotic Clinics* 23(3): 60-61, 1988.

15. Hart L: Lives that are whole. *Life Magazine* 8: 112 December 1988.

16. Radocy B: Voluntary closing control: A successful new design approach to an old concept. *Clinical Prosthetics & Orthotics* 10(2): 82, 1986.

17. Ford C, Grotz RC, Shamp JK: The neurophysiological ankle-foot orthosis. *Clinical Prosthetics & Orthotics* 10(1): 15-23, 1986.

18. Hale S: Carbon fiber articulated AFO—An alternative design. *Journal of Orthotics and Prosthetics* 1(4): 191-198, 1989.

19. Flandry F, Burke S, Roberts JM, Hall S, Drouilhet A, Davis G, Cook S: Functional ambulation in myelodysplasia: The effect of orthotic selection on physical and physiologic performance, *Journal of Pediatric Orthopedics* 6: 661-665, 1986.

20. Hobson DA: Research and development considerations and engineering perspective. *Clinical Prosthetics & Orthotics* 10(4): 122-129, 1986.

Funding for Assistive Technology and Related Services: An Annotated Bibliography

Alexandra Enders

Accent Guide: 151 Tax Deductions You Can Take. G. Thomsen. Accent Special Publications, P.O. Box 700, Bloomington, IL 61701. 1982. 20 pages.

Medical expense deduction guide for individual taxpayers. Especially helpful to those with disabilities. More current information is also available from Internal Revenue Service publications, listed below.

"Adaptive Motor Vehicle Funding," K. Beck. *Paraplegia News*. June 1988, page 14.

Provides a brief overview of the Veteran's Administration adaptive motor vehicle program's funding procedures. This program, with rare exception, is available only to service-connected veterans.

"All Problems Great and Small," R. Howard. *Rx Home Care*. August 1982, pages 38-42.

Suggests four major considerations for dealing effectively with Medicare: clear

Alexandra Enders, OTR, is Research Director at the University of Montana Rehabilitation Technology Center on Rural Rehabilitation, 33 Corbin Hall, Missoula, MT 59812.

Please help us make this resource list more comprehensive. If you know of other materials that should be included, please send information to the author at the address provided above.

Development of this bibliography was begun as part of the activities of the Rehabilitation Technology Service Delivery Project at the Electronic Industries Foundation in Washington, DC, with support in part by Grant No. G008535151 from the National Institute on Disability and Rehabilitation Research, U.S. Department of Education. Continued development is supported by the Institute for Human Resources in Rural America at the University of Montana in Missoula, MT, in part through a Rehabilitation Research and Training Center Grant No. G0087C0228 from the National Institute on Disability and Rehabilitation Research, U.S. Department of Education.

lines of communication with carrier as intermediary; thorough understanding of the regulations and the intermediary's interpretation of the regulations; clear and comprehensive documentation on claims; and effective bill management.

American Journal of Occupational Therapy. May 1984. Special Issue on Reimbursement.

All articles may be of interest. "Medicare: A Summary of Coverage for Occupational Therapy Services, Reimbursement Guidelines, and Covered Durable Medical Equipment" may be of particular interest. This information may be superceded by the 3/88 book from AOTA on reimbursement.

The AOPA Medicare Manual. A. Berriman. American Orthotic and Prosthetic Association. Second Edition. 1981.

A working manual for AOPA members that presents guidelines and regulations, information on determination of reasonable charge, carrier relations, describes the appeals process, reimbursement under Part A. A history of medical assistance is included. The appendices present case studies, and a final report of the Medicare/Government Programs Survey.

"Appealing Medicare Denials," Lori Anderson. *American Journal of Occupational Therapy*, pages 353-358, June, 1988.

Explains the step by step procedures in the Medicare appeals process and gives suggestions for presenting a case so that a denial will have a good chance of being overturned. Presented from the perspective of occupational therapy services, but the process is also applicable to technology and related services.

Applications for Insurance: "Prior Authorization." Prentke Romich Co., 1022 Heyl Road, Wooster, OH 44691. 1987. 11 pages.

Discusses components of process in applying for insurance: materials to be assembled by client advocate, sample letters of support, and how to appeal a denied request.

Applying for Medicaid/PHC/BHC Funding of Communication Devices. P. Fabricant, A. Kraat, C. Schaeffler. December 1983, 22 pages. Available from Carol Schaeffler, UCPA, 1601 Lawrence Ave., Brooklyn, NY 11230.

Prepared for the Funding Committee of Metro-Innovative Communication Alternatives for the Non-Speaking, (Metro I-Can), this paper outlines procedures for applying to Medicaid and the Physically Handicapped Children's program for purchase of communication aids. Covers use of forms, report writing, justification of need, and follow-up strategies if request is denied.

Assistive Financing for Assistive Devices: Loan Guarantees for Purchase of Products by Persons with Disabilities. K. Reeb. January 1989. Electronic Industries Foundation, Rehabilitation Engineering Center, 1901 Pennsylvania Ave., NW, Suite 700, Washington, DC 20006. 29 pages. Free.

Challenges and Rewards: Advocacy for Disability Claimants. $25.00 plus $1.50 postage and handling. Advocates for the Disabled, 4732 South Central Ave., Phoenix, AZ 85040

A how-to workbook and manual on reversing social security disability benefit denials.

Claims Coding Guide: The Wheelchair. 1987. Medicare Part B. Reimbursement. A New York State Blue Cross manual.

Illustrated claims coding guide which identifies various types of wheelchairs and replacement parts for repairs. Includes section on seating and positioning accessories.

Code of Federal Regulations (CFR). Available for sale from: Superintendent of Documents, Government Printing Office, Washington, D.C., 20402. (Most law libraries will have current copies of the CFR and the Federal Register.)

CFR is a codification of the general and permanent rules published in the Federal Register by the Executive departments and the agencies of the Federal Government. The Code is divided into 50 titles which represent broad areas subject to Federal regulation. Each title is divided into chapters which usually bear the name of the issuing agency. Each chapter is further divided into parts covering specific regulatory areas. A complete listing of the CFR Titles and Chapter headings is included in each volume of the series. Titles of particular interest include:

- 20 Employees' Benefits, I Office of Workers' Compensation Programs 20 Employees' Benefits, III Social Security Administration;
- 34 Education, III Office of Special Education and Rehabilitative Services (Special Education Program, Vocational Rehabilitation Program);
- 42 Public Health, IV Heath Care Financing Administration (Medicare and Medicaid Programs).

"Communication Devices Available But Are Out of Reach of Many." *Accent on Living.* Spring 1981, pages 27-35.

Discusses communication devices that have been developed and manufactured and points out difficulties with having items marketed; specifically, training of referring professionals and funding.

"Communication Options for Persons Who Cannot Speak: Planning for Service Delivery," D. Beukelman. 16 pages. *Planning and Implementing Augmentative Communication Service Delivery.* Available through RESNA, 1101 Connecticut Ave. N.W., Suite 700, Washington, D.C., 20036. 1988, 244 pages, $25.00

Paper presented at the National Planners Conference on Assistive Device Service Delivery, Chicago, IL April 1987. Identifies funding issues and makes general recommendations. Deals with variety of funding services, sponsors of augmentative services; public education's responsibility.

Computer Assistance for People with Disabilities. N. Scott. California State University, Northridge, Computer Access Lab, Office of Disabled Student's Service, 18111 Nordhoff Street, Northridge, CA 91330 818/885-2684. 1987. $24.95.

Explores use of computers for assisting people with disabilities. Comprehensive report includes chapter on funding sources and problems. Separately covers funding issues for an individual and for organizations. Also discusses the organization of volunteer programs. Highly recommends *Financing Adaptive Technology* by Steven B. Mendelsohn.

"Creative Funding for Augmentative Communication Services," M. Buzolick, 6 pages. *Planning and Implementing Augmentative Communication Service Delivery.* Available through RESNA, 1101 Connecticut Ave. N.W., Suite 700, Washington, D.C., 20036. 1988, 244 pages, $25.00

Paper presented at the National Planners Conference on Assistive Device Service Delivery, Chicago, IL April 1987. Discusses approaches toward obtaining community funding for non-oral communication services and equipment, and for establishing cooperative effort among various social service agencies to meet needs of client. Outlines strategies for client referral, determination of service and equipment needs, and obtaining necessary funds.

"Creative Funding for Services," M. Buzolick. 5 pages. *Implementation Strategies for Improving the Use of Communication Aids in Schools Serving Handicapped Children.* In press, available from ASHA.

Strategy presented for obtaining community resources for assessment and intervention services to children with severe expressive communication disorders.

"Credit Financing Offered to Wheelchair End-Users," *Homecare*, July 1987, page 86.

Describes the equipment financing programs offered by Everest & Jennings, and Contemporary Health Systems.

"Dealing With Medicare Denials: A Two-Point Strategy," A. Baird and J. Ahl Clark. *Continuing Care.* August 1988, pages 28-29.

Describes an appeals process for home health visits. This approach, although designed for use in Californa, could serve as a model for other areas experiencing routine Medicare denials.

"Determining When DME Can Be Furnished To Long Term Care Facility Residents," E. Carder. *NAMES Resource Section*, Spring 1987, pages 10-11. Insert in *Homecare*. June 1987.

Describes specific statutory and regulatory provisions affecting the determination of Medicare reimbursement for DME for beneficiaries residing in different types of nursing homes.

"Does Your Personal Health Insurance Plan Cover Assistive Technology?"
A. Enders. *Rehabilitation Technology Review.* Winter 1988. pages 1 and 7.

Recommends that all individuals should examine their health insurance coverage for assistive technology. Suggests ways for individuals to have an impact on the reimbursement system.

"Do Products for the Disabled Cost Too Much?" B. Williams. *Accent on Living.* Spring 1979. pages 33-41.

Details factors affecting costs of products for disabled persons: retail mark-up, product liability, insurance and laws, quality control, and government bureaucracy.

"Do Our Payment Policies Encourage Dependency?" K. Reeb. *Proceedings of ICAART, the 1988 RESNA Conference.* Available from RESNA.

"Do You Read, Understand Medicare Carrier Reports?" P. Kraemer. *Homecare.* February 1986, pages 92,95,96.

Stresses the need to pay close attention to, and to follow up on, the "carrier remarks" on disallowed Medicare claims for DME. Interprets some of the commonly used carrier remarks, and what can be done in response.

Do Your Health Insurance Benefits Cover Speech, Language, and Hearing Services? American Speech-Language-Hearing Association, 10801 Rockville, MD 20852

Brochure that covers the basics of examining your health insurance benefits for coverage of a specific type of service. Ideas are applicable to assistive technology and related services.

"DME in Nursing Homes: Exploding the Myth," F. Case. *Washington Report.* Vol. II, No.11. pages 4 and 6. National Association of Medical Equipment Suppliers (NAMES).

Describes how "HCFA has been deliberately and systematically denying coverage of DME to eligible beneficiaries, residents of Intermediate Care Facilities." Also explains the differences between a medicare-certified SNF, a state SNF, an ICF, and an ICF classified as an 1861(j)(1) skilled facility.

DRG Monitor. Hanley & Belfus, Inc., 210 South 13th Street, Philadelphia, PA 19107.

Monthly newsletter reports the key implications of new DRG and Prospective Payment regulations on hospital management.

Durable Medical Equipment: Guidelines for Recommendations for Purchase. State of California, Department of Health Services, California Children Services, 714 P Street, Sacramento, CA 95814, 1985, 10 pages.

Provides guidelines for selection of equipment within "benefits" schedule of

CCS. Charts medical condition and criteria for use of equipment for self-care, mobility, and positioning devices.

Electronic Devices for Rehabilitation. J. Webster et al. John Wiley & Sons, Publishers, New York, NY 1985, 446 pages. $45.00.

In chapter 1: "General Concepts," Al Cook discusses funding of assistive devices and describes the service delivery process.

"Emphasis on Funding," M. Williams. *Proceedings of the Second International Conference on Rehabilitation Engineering.* 1984. Available from RESNA.

Engineering Disability: Public Policy and Compensatory Technology. S. Tannenbaum. Temple University Press, Philadelphia, PA 19122. 1986, 171 pages, $24.95.

Explores social and public policy questions related to the development and distribution process for compensatory technology for disabled people. Provides good descriptions of systems that provide coverage for technology: Veterans' Administration, private and public worker compensation insurance plans, Medicaid, private health insurance.

Enhanced Consumerism within Commercial Rehabilitation Product Markets: A Goal for Independent Living. K. Reeb, Electronic Industries Foundation, Rehabilitation Engineering Center, 1901 Pennsylvania Ave., NW, Suite 700, Washington, DC 20006, January 1986, 37 pages and appendix.

Presents experiences of various service programs on encouragement of more active consumerism by disabled individuals. Support services are classified in the areas of: financing, information collection, training, maintenance/repair, and used equipment exchanges. Group purchase opportunities are explored.

"Ensuring Technology Reaches Those Who Can Benefit By It," A. Enders. Part IV in *Assistive Technology Sourcebook.* 1989. RESNA Press, 1101 Connecticut Ave, N.W. Washington, D.C., 20036.

"Environmental Control Units: Are They Really Luxury Devices?" M. Strait and S. Fridie. *Proceedings of ICAART 88, the 1988 RESNA Conference,* pages 176-177, Available from RESNA.

Describes the need to reassess current reimbursement policies for technology, such as environmental control units, which enhance functional ability.

Evaluation of the Assistive Devices Program: Summary Report to the Advisory Committee on Assistive Devices. B .J. MacDonald and T. Nichols. Ministry of Health, 15 Overlea Blvd., Toronto, Ontario, Canada.

Comprehensive report on the development of the ADP and an evaluation study to determine its effectiveness. Includes research design and results of second study conducted to determine the extent of usage and satisfaction with the assistive devices which were acquired through the ADP. Survey materials and tables of data for each study are presented.

"Expanding Appeal Rights for Medicare Part B Providers: Part 1," "A Practical Guide to the New Part B Appeal Process: Part 2," F. Case and A. Lipsitz. *Homecare*, Part 1, January 1987, pages 46, 48. Part 2, February 1987, pages 90-95.

"Fighting Back," D. Efron. *Homecare*, pages 40-42.
Points out obstacles blocking homecare as a viable source of health care delivery. Recommends use of professional lobbyists to affect legislative change, fight budgetary battles and offset clout of other competitive, lobbying groups.

Final Report of Funding Subcommittee. J. M. Carlson. 7 pages. April 7, 1986. Available from Office of Technology and Disability, Governor's Office of Science and Technology, 150 East Kellogg Blvd., St. Paul, MN 55101.
Discusses issues related to private and public funding sources for rehabilitation technology in Minnesota. Offers specific recommendations concerning redefinition of terminology, loosening of arbitrary bureaucratic procedures, and prior authorization restrictions.

Final Report of the National Task Force on Third Party Payment for Rehabilitation Equipment. K. Reeb. Electronic Industries Foundation, Rehabilitation Engineering Center, 1901 Pennsylvania Ave., NW, Suite 700, Washington, DC 20006, February 1987, 49 pages and appendix.
Discusses issues related to third party payment for rehabilitation equipment and outlines potential strategies for dealing with these problems. Issues include the need for: reliable evaluatory information about rehabilitation products; study of problems related to reimbursement of clinical and technical services that are required for appropriate selection and use of equipment; and improved communication and interaction among all parties involved in use of and payment for equipment. Appendix lists Task Force participants.

"Financial Aid and Special Services," V. Gives. *Disability and Rehabilitation Handbook*. McGraw-Hill, 1978, pages 186-199.
Provides overview of financial aid programs and services available to the disabled individual. Focus is on Social Security, Medicare, Medicaid and public agencies. Also includes private insurance.

Financial Aid for Students with Disabilities. Higher Education and Adult Training for People with Handicaps (HEATH), HEATH Resource Center, One Dupont Circle, N.W., Washington, DC 20036-1193. 800/544-3284 or 800/333-INFO (333-4636).
A regularly updated fact sheet which includes information about funding assistive technology at the post-secondary level.

Financial Aid for the Disabled and Their Families. 1988-1989. Reference Service Press, 10 Twin Dolphin Drive, Suite B-308, Redwood City, CA 94065. 270 pages.

Annotated resource list of scholarships, fellowships, loans, grants, awards and internships designed primarily or exclusively for persons with disabilities and their families. Includes state sources of benefits and reference sources on financial aids.

Financial Resources for Disabled Individuals. Institute for Information Studies, 200 Little Falls Street, Suite 104, Falls Church, VA 22046, 1980, 64 pages and appendices.

Identifies national programs which provide resources for financial benefits to the disabled, and gives qualifying information for each. Organized by interest areas: cash grants, housing, food, health, education, and employment. Also covers general application procedures. Appendices include lists of federal information centers and services.

"Financing Adaptive Aids," *Sensory Aids Technology Update*, December 1983. Available from Sensory Aids Foundation, 399 Sherman Avenue, #12, Palo Alto, CA 94306.

Describes several programs that offer financial aid and/or low interest loans for the purchase of sensory aids for the blind.

Financing Adaptive Technology: A Guide To Sources and Strategies for Blind and Visually Impaired Users. S. Mendelsohn, Smiling Interfaces, P.O. Box 2792, Church Street Station, New York, NY 10008-2792, May 1987, 206 pages, $20.00; specify format: print, braille, audio cassette, Apple IIe disk. Also available through Demos Publications, 156 Fifth Avenue, Suite 108, New York, NY 10010. $24.95.

*Recommended. See book review on last page of bibliography.

Financing Health Care for Handicapped Children: Report of a Workshop. Information Sciences Research Institute, 8027 Leesburg Pike, Suite 102, Vienna, VA 22180. 703/448-1143. 1984, 52 pages.

Provides a good overview of existing programs and problems; offers recommendations for improving availablility of care from all resources: public, private and voluntary.

Financing Sensory Aids. American Foundation for the Blind. 15 West 16th Street, New York, NY 10011. 800/232-5463

Audiotape of a panel discussion on financing sensory aids. It highlights the resource guide written by Steve Mendelsohn, *Financing Adaptive Technology: A Guide To Sources and Strategies for Blind and Visually Impaired Users*. Available directly from AFB, National Technology Center.

"Forms That Make Insurers Pay Up," C. Irvin, J.D., *Medical Economics*. January 24, 1983, pages 118-120.

Describes sample forms for collecting patient information, and for uncovering the reasons third party payers have not paid the charges. Makes suggestions for using forms to get full benefits from the patient's insurance coverage and to challenge insurance carriers' underpayments.

"Funding," Chapter 5. *The Resource Manual. Second Edition*. The Carroll Center for the Blind, Computer Access for the Blind in Education and Employment (CABLE) Project, 770 Centre Street, Newton, MA 02158. $25.00.

"Funding and Service Delivery of Augmentative Communication Devices in Ontario, Canada: Status and Issues," P. Parnes. 9 pages and appendices, *Planning and Implementing Augmentative Communication Service Delivery*. Available through RESNA, 1101 Connecticut Ave. N.W., Suite 700, Washington, D.C., 20036. 1988, 244 pages, $25.00

Paper presented at the National Planners Conference on Assistive Device Service Delivery, Chicago, IL, April 1987. Details delivery service of augmentative communication devices in Ontario. System closely links service delivery with provision of devices through development of a system of clinics and clinic levels. Model includes provision of equipment leasing rather than purchase. Outlines strengths and weaknesses as system now operates.

"Funding Assistive Devices," *PAM Repeater, No. 42: Funding Resources*, September 1987, 24 pages. $2.00. Available from PAM Assistance Centre, 601 West Maple Street, Lansing, MI 48906

Describes assistive technology funding resources available in Michigan. Lists agencies in order by organizational categories which are sources of assistive devices or funding. Briefly discusses the process of applying for funding, includes generic suggestions for obtaining funding, a Personal Information Data Sheet, and other basic material useful for other states.

"Funding Assistive Devices Services and Individual Equipment," R. Dodds. 9 pages, *Planning and Implementing Augmentative Communication Service Delivery*. Available through RESNA, 1101 Connecticut Ave. N.W., Suite 700, Washington, D.C., 20036. 1988, 244 pages, $25.00

Paper presented at the National Planners Conference on Assistive Device Service Delivery, Chicago, IL April 1987. Provides guidelines for obtaining funds to establish Assistive Device Centers; includes outline for development of funding proposals for services, and guidelines for acquiring funds to purchase equipment. Lists federal and private funding agencies.

"Funding Challenges," M. Williams. *Seating for Children with Cerebral Palsy*, pages 181-183. University of Tennessee Rehabilitation Engineering Program, 682 Court, Memphis, TN, 1984.

Discusses funding issues as they relate to the University of Tennessee Rehabilitation Engineering Program. Points out need for establishing an adequate, secure funding base.

Funding Devices and Services in Augmentative and Alternative Communication. Prentke Romich Company, 1022 Heyl Road, Wooster, OH 44691; 800/642-8255.
Poster that depicts a wide range of available funding options. Also available as a wall chart.

"Funding for Augmentative Communication Aids," P. Johnston. *Express Yourself*, pages 111-138. Pegijohn, 6432 Fifth Avenue South, Richfield, MN 55423 $9.95 + $2.00 postage.

"Funding High Tech: Insurmountable Hurdle or Just a Matter of Hard Work?" *Computer Disability News*. Winter 87/88. National Easter Society, Chicago, IL.
Interview with Carol Cohen, Director of the Adaptive Services Division, UCPA, Syracuse, NY.

"Funding: How You Can Make It Work," Anna Hoffman. 14 pages. *Planning and Implementing Augmentative Communication Service Delivery*. Available through RESNA, 1101 Connecticut Ave. N.W., Suite 700, Washington, D.C., 20036. 1988, 244 pages, $25.00
Paper presented at the National Planners Conference on Assistive Device Service Delivery, Chicago, IL, April 1987. Presents overview of legislative history and federal studies in past decade concerning the physically disabled. Points out need for continued work in advocacy toward further study and funding. Also explores strategies for obtaining funding. Focuses on need for check-list; appropriate wording on claim, advantages of appealing denials. Includes sample check-list.

"Funding, Models, Policy, Statistics," A. Enders. Chapter 8. *Technology for Independent Living Sourcebook*. 1984. RESNA.

Funding of Mobility Equipment: Current Issues and Strategies. V. Ruggles, Muscular Dystrophy Association, 810 Seventh Avenue, New York, NY 10019, 1981, 13 pages and appendices.
Outlines procedure for securing funds for mobility equipment. Lists and describes funding sources. Discusses advocacy issues.

Funding of Non Vocal Communication Aids: Current Issues and Strategies. V. Ruggles, Muscular Dystrophy Association, 810 Seventh Avenue, New York, NY 10019, 30 pages.
Outlines procedure for securing funds for communication equipment. Lists and describes funding sources. Discusses advocacy issues.

Funding Panel Videotape. Tape can be borrowed from Disabled Children's Computer Group, 2095 Rose Street, Berkeley, California.

Amateur-produced tape of a presentation to parents and professionals on 9/17/87 about funding for computer-based equipment.

"Funding Sources and Strategies," K. Reeb and S. McFarland. *Rehabilitation Technology Service Delivery: A Practical Guide*, Chapter 5, pages 107-123. RESNA. 1988. 175 pages. $18.00.

Chapter deals with three central issues for rehabilitation technology service delivery: the funds to start a business, the capabilities that will earn money, and the needs for which payers will spend their funds. Profiles various third party payment programs, including Medicare, Medicaid, Vocational Rehabilitation and the private insurance system.

Funding Strategies for the 1980s: Report of the Advanced Topical Discussion, Aug. 22, 1982. A. Enders. May 1983. Available from author, through RESNA.

Explains some of the major obstacles to funding, and the strategies that have been successful in obtaining funding.

"Funding Technology Devices: Ways Through the Maze," H. Pressman. *Exceptional Parent*. October 1987, pages 48-52.

Points out various considerations to take into account for successful funding applications.

Funding: The Bottom Line. A. Enders. 1983. 8 pages (expanded version of a paper by the same name in the 1983 RESNA proceedings), available from author, through RESNA.

Focuses on funding issues concerned with third party reimbursement in the public sector. Provides an outline describing steps in the funding process.

"Funding VOCAs for the Lower Cognitive Functioning Population," G. Turner. Page 26. *Closing the Gap*. December 1986/January 1987.

Describes complexity of obtaining funding for this population, and relates success in securing funding for voice output communication aids through Section 55 of Michigan's State Aid to Education Bill.

"General Concepts," A. Cook. *Electronic Devices for Rehabilitation*, Chapter 1, pages 3-30. John Wiley and Sons, 1985.

Discusses types and systems of funding for electronic assistive devices and services.

A Guide to Medical Assistance Plans (Medicaid). American Orthotic and Prosthetic Association. 1981. 6 volumes.

Comprehensive review of Medicaid coverage, and summary of individual state plans in regard to orthotics, prosthetics, as well as a range of durable medical equipment. States are grouped by regions.

A Guide to Rehabilitation. P. Deutsch and H. Sawyer. Mathew Bender, publishers. 1986.
A guide for rehabilitation professionals working with injured or disabled workers.

Guidelines for Seeking Funding for Communication Aids. D. DePape. Revised 1988. 7 pages and 21 pages of appendices. Trace Center, 1500 Highland Drive, University of Wisconsin, Madison, WI 53705.
Provides guidelines to assist in organizing plans to obtain funding for purchase of communication aids. Appendices include listings of possible funding sources, state service agencies, state vocation rehabilitation agencies, and directories of same.

Handicapped Funding Directory. 1986-87 Fifth Edition. R. Eckstein. Research Grant Guides, P.O.Box 10726, Marina del Ray, CA 90726. 194 pages. $23.50.
Lists over 700 foundations, corporations, government agencies and associations which grant funds to institutions and agencies for handicapped programs and services. Oriented to obtaining program funding rather than grants to individuals. Even with the book, further research through one of the Foundation Center collections is usually necessary.

"**Handicapped Independence Assistance Act of 1983**," transcript in *Congressional Record* – Senate, April 20, 1983.
Transcript of Senator Matsunaga's bill S.1115, to treat certain sensory and communication aids as medical and other health services. The bill did not become a law, but its existence should be noted.

"**HCFA 1500: Dealers Learn To Get It Right at HIDA Seminar**," *Homecare*, October 1987, page 20.
Tips for completing HCFA-1500 claims forms are given. Excerpted from one of the Health Industry Distributors Association's Clean Claims Seminars.

HCPCS Codes: Listing and Medicare Billing Guide. California Association of Medical Product Suppliers (CAMPS). 1987. 38 pages. $34.95, plus $3.00 for shipping and handling. Available from: CAMPS, 660 J Street, Suite 480, Sacramento, CA 95814.
Using the correct billing code is a major part of expediting reimbursement. A list of nearly 90 percent of the most commonly used Health Care Procedure Codes (HCPC) have been matched to manufacturer's products in an effort by one state association to help end home medical equipment (HME) dealer confusion over Medicare reimbursement codes. It is believed that using the guide will allow dealers to cut down on the medical review process and speed up reimbursement payments by billing by specific code, rather than relying on miscellaneous codes. The

guide also contains comparisons to selected non-Medicare codes and useful Medicare requirements, including basic prescription requirements, billing modifiers, and fraud and abuse guidelines.

Health Care and Finances: A Guide for Adult Children and Their Parents. S. Abbott. American Council of Life Insurance and Health Insurance Association of America, 1001 Pennsylvania Avenue, N.W. Washington, D.C., 20004. December, 1987. 21 pages
Identifies some common problems, raises questions and presents some answers about financial planning related to health care.

"Health Care: Who Pays the Bills," M. Morris. *Exceptional Parent.* July 1987, pages 38-42.
Edited version of testimony before the Senate Select Committee on Children, Youth and Families. Includes information on cost differentials for ablebodied and disabled children, including specialized equipment costs.

Home Health Care, Jay Portnow, editor. Physical Medicine and Rehabilitation: State of the Art Reviews, Volume 2, Issue 3. Hanley & Belfus, Inc. 210 South 13th Street, Philadelphia, PA 19107 215/546-7293. 1988, Hardcover, $12.00.
Described as "a practical handbook for home health care professionals," this book includes two chapters on assistive technology, "Self-Help Devices" by Valerie Takai, and "High Technology at Home," by Ruth Dickey. Also includes a chapter on "Reimbursement Issues."

Home Health Care: A Consumer Guide. Illinois Council of Home Health Services. 1985. 15 pages.
Pamphlet providing guidance in the consideration of using home health care, including supportive equipment. Lists available services, and financial information. Written for Illinois, could provide a model for other regions writing resource guides.

"How Can We Pay For All This?" J. Coombs. *Living With the Disabled: You Can Help.* Chapter 7, pages 111-141. Sterling Publishing. 1984.
Covers a broad range of payment sources for disability-related expenses.

How to Beat the High Cost of Learning: The Complete and Up-to-Date Guide to Student Financial Aid. L. Kornfeld, C. Siegel, and W. Seigel, W. Ranson, Wade Publishers, Inc., New York. 1981.
Has a section on Special Students which includes a discussion of students with disabilities.

"How to Collect Everything Third Parties Owe You," A. Owens. *Medical Economics.* August 8, 1983, pages 98-104.
Pointers and practical tips for submitting and following up on claims. Article is based on the observations of physicians, their insurance clerks, medical manage-

ment consultants, and insurance company employees experienced in processing medical claims.

"How to Get Government Money and Other Help," *A Handbook for the Disabled*, S. Lunt. Chapter 28, pages 223-233, Charles Scribner & Sons, 1982.
Lists and describes some of the public and private organizations that can help with financial and other problems encountered by disabled persons. Covers general, self-help, housing, tax, student loans and co-op sources.

How To Obtain Funding for Augmentative Communication Devices. Prentke Romich Company, 1022 Heyl Road, Wooster, OH 44691, 800/642-8255. Revised, 2/89. 24 pages plus sample forms. No charge.
*****Recommended.** Produced by a manufacturer of communication devices, this manual is generic to all communication devices. The information can also be generalized to other types of assistive devices. Primarily oriented toward medically-based funding sources (Medicaid, private health insurance). Includes sections on basic terms, funding options, steps for success in funding, components of a medically-based request, medical necessity, outlines for letters, sample letters, supportive letter request forms, communication prosthesis payment review summary.

"How to Raise Funds for a Good Cause: Success Stories," *Sunset*. pages 158-163.
Not specifically disability oriented, but describes sixteen fund-raising projects and outlines steps for planning a successful fund-raiser.

"If Federal Grants are Cut Back or Eliminated . . . Could Disabled Use Vouchers and Get Better Services?" E. C. Ross. *Accent on Living*. Spring 1982, pages 118-121.
Reviews history of voucher proposals made by various federal agencies to replace certain existing programs for assistance to the disabled population. Presents advantages and disadvantages of such programs and urges readers to contact congressional representatives regarding their views.

The Implications of Cost-Effectiveness Analysis of Medical Technology. Chapter One: "Summary and Policy Options," pages 3-13. U.S. Congress Office of Technology Assessment. Washington, DC.
Outlines options that relate to the current possibilities for using CEA/CBA in policy formulation and decision making and those that relate to the development of CEA/CBA technique in themselves. Study stresses that decision making cannot be done solely on the basis of CEA/CBA, and that other issues must be considered. Good reference when the need to justify going beyond simple CEA data is needed.

"Industry Experts Analyze New Medicare Reimbursement Law," A.Segedy. *Homecare*. February 1988, pages 84-93.

First of a series of articles that interpret implementation procedures for new Medicare reimbursement regulations for durable medical equipment. Included is Subpart B of the Omnibus Budget Reconciliation Act of 1987. In effect, it is the Six-Point Plan as negotiated by the home medical equipment industry lobbyists, Congress and the Reagan administration.

"Insurance Can Help Pay for Adaptive Equipment," G. Robison. *The Exceptional Parent*. May 1986, pages 11-15.

The author, the parent of a disabled child, explains how to approach obtaining insurance funding. Information provided was useful in obtaining an Apple IIe computer-generated Echo II Speech Synthesizer with Unicorn Expanded Keyboard, and a Fortress Scientific Power Wheelchair with special controls for a five-year-old with cerebral palsy.

"Information and Funding for the Speech Impaired," *Health Technology Case Study 26: Assistive Devices for Severe Speech Impairments*, pages 33-45. U.S. Congress, Office of Technology Assessment, Washington, DC, December 1983.

Explores issues related to third party payment for assistive communication devices. Points out industry's problems with reimbursement, particularly for products which are innovative, redesigned, or "orphan." Lists public and private funding programs.

"Insurance Reimbursement and the Physical Therapist," *Clinical Management and Physical Therapy*. March/April 1987, Special Section, pages 21-40.

Articles in this section are designed to aid practitioners in understanding and dealing with insurance reimbursement. Includes a glossary, claims processing tips, a guide to filing insurance claims, and information on documentation.

Internal Revenue Service Publications. Available from District IRS offices, or calling 800/424-FORM. (800/424-3676)

Information about tax credits and deductions can be found in:

- #17 Your Federal Income Tax.
- #502 Deductions for Medical and Dental Expenses.
- #503 Child Care and Disabled Dependent Care.
- #907 Tax Information for Handicapped and Disabled Individuals

"IRS Lists Additional Tax Exemptions for Disabled," *Mainstream*. January 1983, pages 26-27.

Reports some of the deductions allowed as medical expense on federal income tax and points out the need to substantiate deductions itemized on tax returns. (See more current information from IRS.)

Loans for Accessibility and related material, The Corporation for Independent Living, 30 Jordan Lane, Wethersfield, CT 06109.

Describes Connecticut state-wide low-interest loan program designed for low or moderate income people who are physically disabled to modify their existing housing. (This program and others are also described in Reeb's *Revolving Loan Funds: Expanding Equipment Credit Financing Opportunities for Persons with Disabilities.*)

"Long Term Care: How to develop and write better restorative care plans." *Common Problems, Useful Solutions*, Vol.2, No.3, 1989, 40 pages, $1.50. Ali Med, 297 High Street, Dedham, MA 02026, 800/225-2610.

*Recommended. A catalog of AliMed products written descriptively from the functional perspective of the measurable outcome that a restorative care product will provide. Organized into problem areas in activities of daily living, skin care, and wheelchair seating and positioning. Products that have been used successfully in solving problems are presented along with selection criteria. For each type of problem there is a problem statement, a goal statement and a restorative care plan. It states that you can "use, adapt or copy this material as it is helpful in your facility." If more catalogs were written like this one, it would be easier for practitioners to select appropriate equipment, and to compose succinct outcome-oriented funding justifications. A catalog in this format is a creative approach to marketing, but it also provides a real service. The manufacturer clearly understands the problems in his market. He has found a way to help practitioners do a better job, and to sell his products at the same time.

Making the Most of Medicare. Arthur Pell. Prentice Hall. 1987. $10.95.

Many Faces of Funding, Anna Hoffman, Phonic Ear, Inc., 250 Camino Alto, Mill Valley, CA 94941. Binder with updates is $35.00, Newsletter is $5.00/year.
*Recommended. Produced by a manufacturer of communication devices. Discusses major third-party funding programs including federal/state, educational, insurance and private funding sources. Outlines comprehensive procedure for application and describes case histories. Updated monthly with Newsletter. Although targeted toward communication devices, this material is useful generically to anyone developing funding strategies for assistive devices.

"Maximizing Reimbursement from Managed Care Organizations," M. Reber. *Rx Home Care*. April 1987, pages 37-38.
Cautions dealers of DME items concerning issues related to HMO contracting.

Medical Screening List for Durable Medical Equipment. Abbey Medical.
Lists durable medical equipment and their coverage status under Medicare.

Medicaid/Medical Assistance Program Provider Manuals.
Will generally contain basic information concerning the submission and processing of claims. Look for this type of information through the organization in your state that administers the medicaid/medical assistance program.

"Medicaid Reimbursement for Rehabilitation Equipment: Overview," A. Markowitz and K. Reeb. *Assistive Technology.* Vol.1, #1, 1989. pages 11-17. (*Assistive Technology* is the official journal of RESNA. It is available through Demos Publications, 156 Fifth Avenue, Suite 108, New York, NY 10010.)

Based on a telephone survey done in late 1987 by the Electronic Industries Foundation Rehabilitation Engineering Center, this report documents current Medicaid coverage for assistive technology. It also analyzes some of the general policies and practices of the Medicaid system as they relate to assistive technology.

Medicare Carriers Manual. Section on Claims Processing. Health Care Financing Administration, U.S. Department of Health and Human Services, Washington, DC. October 1986. Updates available only through subscription, $200.00 + / year.

Sections of the Medicare Carriers Manual cover prosthetic devices and durable medical equipment and their coverage status.

Medicare Made Easy. C. Inlander, C. MacKay. Addison-Wesley Publishing Company, Jacob Way, Reading, MA 01867. 1989, 336 pages, $10.95.

Produced by the People's Medical Society, takes an advocacy approach. Includes information on the Medicare Catastrophic Coverage Act; samples of forms, with full explanations; how to negotiate fees; how to select supplemental insurance; and strategies for making Medicare work for you.

"Medicare/Medicaid Home Care Product Reimbursement — A Chronology," M. Vranizan. *Homecare.* March 1987, page 26.

Briefly describes the changes in reimbursement from 1965 to 1987.

"Medicare Part B and the Appeals Process," A. Erenberg. *Continuing Care Coordinator.* February 1985, pages 6 and 28.

Outlines steps to take in appealing Medicare Part B payment decisions.

"Medicare Part B Appeals: Strategies for Fair Hearings, Judicial Review," E. Carder. *Homecare.* November 1986, pages 156-160.

Changes in the appeals process, and the newly available judicial review process are explained. Article focuses on helping "DME dealers understand their appeal rights and how they can best exercise them."

"Medicare's Growing Pains," A. Berriman. *AOPA Almanac.* October 1985, pages 22-23.

Brief history of Medicare's evolvement since its inception in 1965.

"A New Concept of Subsidy in Determining Fees for Service," A.Goldberg and D. Kovac. *Social Casework.* April 1971, pages 206-210. **"Implementing a Fee System Based On Appropriate Subsidy"** A. Goldberg and D. Kovac. *Social Casework.* April 1973, pages 233-238.

These articles present a different perspective on subsidized fee for service structures. Read them in conjunction with Reeb's paper on *Revolving Loan Funds*, listed below, if you are interested in encouraging the agencies you work with to develop alternative private payment strategies.

New Tax Code Changes Will Clarify Deductible Expenses for Access Modifications. A. Virellas. Paralyzed Veterans of America, 1801 H Street, Washington, DC, 4 pages.

Describes allowable tax deductions under the Tax Reform Act of 1986.

The Non-Oral Communication Panel in Contra Costa County. R. Hansen. 4 pages. UCPA.

Defines the Non-Oral Communication Panel and its role in designing and providing non-oral communication systems for clients in Contra Costa County, CA.

"Obtaining Insurance Funding for Your Handicapped Dependents Needs," G. Robison and A. Robison. *Communication Outlook.* Winter 1985, pages 7-8.

Describes an action plan and the sequence of events necessary for obtaining funding for assistive technology from an insurance company.

"An Outreach Program: Addressing the Needs of the Physically Impaired in Rural Communities," E. Moore and D. Allen. *Planning and Implementing Augmentative Communication Service Delivery.* Available through RESNA, 1101 Connecticut Ave. N.W., Suite 700, Washington, DC 20036. 1988, 244 pages, $25.00.

Paper presented at the National Planners Conference on Assistive Device Service Delivery, Chicago, IL, April 1987.

"Overcoming Obstacles to Medicaid Reimbursement," B. Leyrer. *Rx Homecare.* January 1987.

Written from the Medicaid agency's perspective. Emphasizes need for consumers, vendors and providers to cultivate relationships with agency decision makers. Stresses that better communication results in better payment decisions.

"Paying for the Medical Help You Need," M. Jones. *Home Care for the Chronically Ill or Disabled Child.* Harper & Row. 1985.

Presents an advocacy-oriented approach to finding the resources you need. The author is the parent of a disabled child, and understands the complexities of the process.

"Paying for the Stuff," S. Mendelsohn. *Technology Update.* Sensory Aids Foundation, 399 Sherman, Palo Alto, CA.

Starting with the December 1987 issue, Steve Mendelsohn is writing a regular column on financing assistive technology.

Payment for Assistive Devices by the Veterans Administration. K. Reeb.

Electronic Industries Foundation, 1901 Pennsylvania Avenue, #700, Washington, DC 20006. March 1989.

Payment for Occupational Therapy Services. American Occupational Therapy Association, 1383 Piccard, Rockville, MD. March 1988. $50 members, $65 nonmembers.

Details existing coverage for O.T. services within state, federal and private payment systems. Includes information on documentation, billing and durable medical equipment.

"Payment Issues and Options in the Utilization of Assistive Technology," Steven Mendelsohn. Pages 94-118 in *Provision of Assistive Technology: Planning and Implementation, Report of a Workshop, March 8-10, 1989.* Electronic Industries Foundation, 1901 Pennsylvania Avenue, NW, Suite 700, Washington, DC 20006.

Payment Refused. William Shernoff. Richardson and Steirman, publishers.

Written by a California lawyer, book describes fighting insurance companies in court and winning.

"Perspectives on Funding," C. Cohen. 6 pages. *Planning and Implementing Augmentative Communication Service Delivery.* Available through RESNA, 1101 Connecticut Ave. N.W., Suite 700, Washington, DC 20036. 1988, 244 pages, $25.00.

Paper presented at the National Planners Conference on Assistive Device Service Delivery, Chicago, IL, April 1987. Identifies four components of funding process: supporting the diagnostic evaluation site; client-assessment and training; client-owned and operated systems; research and product design. Presents and details Schneier Communication Unit Funding Model (UCP) as a successful approach to procuring funds.

Pictorial Reference Manual of Orthotics and Prosthetics. American Orthotic and Prosthetic Association. 1986. 250 pages.

Provides generic illustrations and brief descriptions of procedures and devices used in orthotics-prosthetics.

Planning and Implementing Augmentative Communication Service Delivery, C. Costen, editor. Available from RESNA, 1101 Connecticut Ave. N.W., Suite 700, Washington, DC 20036. 1988, 244 pages, $25.00.

Proceedings of the National Planners Conference on Assistive Device Service Delivery, Chicago, IL, April 1987. Some of the individual papers from this document are also individually referenced in this bibliography. Although the book's emphasis is on communication services, the presenters provide a good overview of the issues in assistive technology service delivery in special education, including funding issues.

Pocket Guide to Federal Help for Individuals with Disabilities. U.S. Department of Education, Clearinghouse on the Handicapped. September 1987, 26 page pamphlet. Available from Government Printing Office, Washington DC GPO # 1987 0 – 192-796 : QL 3.

Provides basic information on principal federal assistance programs available to eligible persons with disabilities.

Preparing for the Six Point Plan. National Association of Medical Equipment Suppliers (NAMES) 625 Slaters Lane, Suite 200, Alexandria, VA 22314, 703/ 836-6263. Two volumes. 1989. $25.00/volume, $45.00/set. Nonmember price is $85.00/set, or $50.00/volume.

Provides durable medical equipment dealers with detailed information, including carrier instructions on reimbursement procedures under Medicare's new Six-Point Plan.

Principles of Reimbursement in Health Care. D. Beck. Aspen Systems. 1983. 293 pages. $41.95.

Written by an accountant with experience in hospital finances, the book is oriented to health care accounting; however, some of the principles may be useful for developing strategies to maximize third party reimbursement.

Private Insurance Reimbursement for Rehabilitation Equipment. K. Reeb. Electronic Industries Foundation, Rehabilitation Engineering Center, 1901 Pennsylvania Ave., NW, Suite 700, Washington, DC 20006, July 1987, 17 pages and bibliography.

Provides a basic understanding of private insurance by defining the fundamental aspects of insurance – what it is and why it exists; discussing the insurance payment process; treating factors involved in payment decision making; and outlining four major policy categories: health insurance, disability insurance, workers' compensation, liability insurance.

Procurement of Durable Medical Equipment Under the Medicare Part B Program. K. Reeb. May 1985. 22 pages and bibliography. Electronic Industries Foundation, Rehabilitation Engineering Center, 1901 Pennsylvania Ave., NW, Suite 700, Washington, DC 20006.

Explains Medicare Part B Program, with particular emphasis on coverage for the rental or purchase of durable medical equipment. Covers maintenance/repair issues. Tables detail equipment and coverage.

Provision of Low Incidence Material for Eligible Special Education Students. Memorandum #10, December 15, 1986. Los Angeles Unified School District. Los Angeles, CA.

Provides definitions, eligbility criteria and procedures for the provision of low incidence material, including assistive technology for special education students in the Los Angeles Unified School District.

"Psychological Damage of Medicare Denial," F. Ward. *Physical Therapy Forum.* April 1, 1987, pages 1,3,4.
Not specifically related to equipment denial. The article raises another aspect of the challenge of finding appropriate support for individuals. Stresses the issue of the client being in control of their life.

Rehabilitation Engineering—A Possible Solution. K. Roy. 6 pages. UCPA Governmental Activities Office, Washington DC.
Suggests possible funding sources for programs which would expand the application of rehabilitation engineering to employment environments and problems.

Rehabilitation of Workers' Compensation and Other Insurance Claimants: Case Management, Forensic and Business Aspects. J. Rasch. Charles C Thomas Publishers, Springfield, IL, 1985. 213 pages.
Part I. Foundations of Private Sector Rehabilitation provides a good overview of the insurance industry and workers'compensation system.

Reimbursement Advisor. E. Metheny, ed. Aspen Publishers. Monthly, 8 pages. $127/year.
Current information on the effects of DRGs and prospective payment system.

"Remedies for Reimbursement Run-ins," M. Hamilton. *Rx Home Care.* April 1987, pages 32-35.
Identifies possible reimbursement problems DME suppliers may encounter and recommends procedures for remedy. This article is part of a special section on Reimbursement.

A Review and Analysis of the "Job Training Partnership Act." President's Committee on Employment of the Handicapped. 16 pages.
Reviews and analyzes the Job Training Partnership Act as it relates, in particular, to handicapped individuals who are economically disadvantaged.

Revolving Loan Funds: Expanding Equipment Credit Financing Opportunities for Persons with Disabilities. K. Reeb. Electronic Industries Foundation, Rehabilitation Engineering Center, 1901 Pennsylvania Ave., NW,C2 Suite 700, Washington, DC 20006, June 1987, 47 pages and appendices.
Comprehensive guide for planning and implementing a revolving loan fund program. Covers program design, pricing of service, establishing fund, and marketing of service. Also explains loan guarantee funds. Tables include decision making checklists, list of medical programs studied, and sample loan forms.

San Francisco Bay Area Occupational Therapy Handbook on Reimbursement. Bay Area Occupational Therapy Forum, 131 Coquito Court, Portola Valley, CA 94025. 1983. $22.00.
Although the data is specific to northern California, and somewhat out of date,

the handbook presents a model for other regions preparing materials relevant to their own reimbursement issues.

Saving Money and Getting Help: Advice for Families of Children With Spina Bifida. L. Rosenfeld, G. Worley, J. Lipscomb. 1987. Spina Bifida Association of N.C., 1427 Robin Lane, Newton, NC 28658. $8.50.
  Practical advice for any family with a disabled child. Includes information on health care insurance coverage. A brief article was reprinted in the November/December 1987 issue of *Exceptional Parent.*

"Service Delivery Systems: Administrative and Clinical Issues in Augmentative Communication," C. Cohen, J. Frumkin. *Seminars in Speech and Language.* May 1987, pages 125-141.
  Describes the development of service delivery systems, the role of the speech and language pathologist, models for service provision, and administrative issues, including funding issues that must be considered.

"The Search for Funding: Providing Justification," A. Bergen. *Homecare.*

Social Security, Medicare and Pensions: An Essential Sourcebook for Older Americans and Their Families. Fourth Edition. J. Mathews. Nolo Press, 950 Parker Street, Berkeley, CA 94710, 415/549-1976. November 1988, $15.95.
  Includes the new Medicare Catastrophic Coverage Act, and a free subscription to Nolo News that contains update info.

"Speech Prosthesis as a Legal Entitlement," R. L. Justice and T. Vogel. *Communication Outlook.* September 1981, pages 8-9.
  Recommends use of a litigation lawyer to overturn denials for assistance. Outlines process for retaining a lawyer, payment consideration, and procedural steps a lawyer may take.

Stalking the Elusive Buck. K. McGuiness. Adaptive Environments Center, Massachusetts College of Art, 621 Huntington Ave, Boston MA 02215. 1982. 65 pages, $5.00.
  Emphasizes funding sources for adapting environments, with an orientation toward resources available in Massachusetts, but the information and recommended approach are generic. Tends toward finding program-oriented funding, but has sections on "Strategies For Applying As An Individual," and "Money For Me." Rules of thumb apply to individuals or non-profit organizations.

Suggested Approach for Establishing A Rehabilitation Engineering Information Service for the State of California. Lo Christy et al. SRI International, 1978. 269 pages, appendices.
  Report of study designed to improve the delivery of services and assistive devices to the disabled by creating a communication network and an improved sys-

tem of information retrieval and dissemination in the rehabilitation community of California. Recommendations made on issues related to funding.

Suggested Procedures for Seeking Funding for Communication Devices. United Cerebral Palsy Association of California. 1982. 3 pages.

Report on findings of a Work Group on Communication Device Funding convened by UCPA of California which gives practical suggestions for obtaining funds.

Tax Information for Handicapped and Disabled Individuals. Department of the Treasury, Internal Revenue Service. Publication 907. Free.

Published annually by the IRS for use in preparing federal income tax returns. Includes information on taxable and non-taxable income items, credit for the elderly or for the permanently and totally disabled, medical expenses, child and dependent car credit, and business tax incentives.

"Tax Reform Followup—What's New for 1989," Heidi Heuple. *Paraplegia News*, January 1989, pages 21-23.

Explains tax provision changes that affect individuals with disabilities.

Team Assessment of Device Effectiveness. J. Kohn et al. Rehabilitation Engineering Center, Children's Hospital at Stanford, Palo Alto, California. 1980.

Describes a study of mobility device effectiveness that includes cost and time factors, as well as an analysis of payment sources for the equipment.

Technology-Dependent Children's Access to Medicaid Home Care Financing. H. Fox and R. Yoshpe. 1986. 47 pages. $13.50. Fox Health Policy Consultants, 1140 Connecticut Ave.N.W., Washington, DC 20036.

Report examines the opportunities that technology-dependent children have for obtaining home care coverage under the Medicaid program.

Technology-Dependent Children: Hospital v. Home Care. A Technical Memorandum. Office of Technology Assessment, U.S. Congress, Washington, DC, May 1987.

Technology and Aging in America. Office of Technology Assessment, U.S. Congress, Washington, DC. Summary available from OTA, full report available from: Government Printing Office, Washington, DC, June, 1985, 496 pages.

An excellent analysis; however, when policy issues and options recommended here are compared to those in OTA's study of technology and disabled people (see citation below), some subtle but substantial discrepancies appear. Because issues related to aging "drive" many of the public policy areas, especially those related to health care reimbursement, it is important to analyze these two sets of policy recommendations in tandem.

Technology and Handicapped People. U.S. Congress Office of Technology

Assessment (OTA). 600 Pennsylvania Ave, S.E., Washington, DC 20510. Summary available from: OTA. Full report available from: S/N 052-003-00874, Superintendent of Documents, Government Printing Office, Washington, DC 20402. 1982, 214 pages. $7.00.

*Recommended. This is an excellent analysis of the entire field of applied technology for disabled people. It examines specific factors that affect the research and development, evaluation, diffusion and marketing, delivery, use and financing of technologies.

Chapter 9, "Delivery, Use and Financing of Technologies," provides a good overview of funding programs and issues. The OTA is currently preparing a 40-50 page update of this document. It should be available in mid-1988, directly from OTA.

"The Therapist's Role in Improving the Person-Environment Fit," D. Olin. *Topics in Geriatric Rehabilitation*, October,1987, pages 43-47.

*Recommended. Provides information on problems obtaining equipment reimbursement and on effective reimbursement strategies. Includes a good example of language that could be used in an equipment justification for a wheelchair.

Third Party Financing of Low Vision Services: A National Study. C. Kirchner. American Foundation for the Blind. Prepared for the National Center for Health Services Research. October 1984. 205 pages. Available from NTIS. Document # PB85 16 432 5. $25.95.

Full report of the study noted below.

"Third Party Financing of Low Vision Services: Pts. 1 and 2," C. Kirchner. *Journal of Visual Impairment and Blindness*, October 1984; February 1985. Statistical Briefs # 29,30. 8 pages.

Presents design of, and results from a study by the American Federation for the Blind, of third party payment for low vision services. Specifically discusses Medicaid and Group Health Insurance (S.B. #29); and State Vocational Rehabilitation Agencies and Low Vision Clinics (S.B. #30).

"Third Party Payer Response to Requests for Purchase of Communication Augmentation Systems: A Study of Washington State," D. Beulelman et al. *AAC Augmentative and Alternative Communication*. February 1985.

Based on a study conducted June 1979-December 1981.

"Time to Slay the Dragon," M. Grant. *Accent on Living*. Spring 1988, pages 104-109.

Describes how one individual fought the system to win financial assistance from SSDI. Includes basic guidelines on how to deal with your social security claim.

"Tips on How to Get Tough With a Soft Touch Help in Collections," *Homecare*. August 1987, pages 24-26.

Describes leading reasons for rejection of patient billing claims. Lists key points to look for in selecting a collection agency, and provides tips for working with consumers before turning bills over to a collection agency.

"Trends in Home Health Care," J. Raymond, *Rehabilitation Gazette*, Vol. 25, 1982, pages 42-44.

Details coverage available under the Home and Community Based Waiver (Title XIX Medicaid Waiver). Also reports on findings of the Surgeon General's Workshop on Children with Handicaps and their Families, and on the Brook Lodge Symposium.

Understanding the Prospective Payment System: A Business Perspective. C. Baum and A. Luebben. Current Practice Series in Occupational Therapy, Vol. 1, No. 1, Slack Inc. 1986. 100 pages.

Describes the Prospective Payment System for Medicare, and its impact on inpatient hospital services. Includes extensive discussion of management skills to enhance hospital function and productivity.

Urgent II. Health Industry Distributors Association (HIDA), 1701 Pennsylvania Avenue NW, Washington, DC 20006, 202/659-0050. 1989. $25.00.

A technical assistance kit dealing with the Medicare's Six-Point Plan for reimbursement of durable medical equipment. Intended to assist the durable medical equipment dealer in expediting claims.

Used Equipment Marketplace: A Strategy for Cutting Equipment Costs. Metropolitan Center for Independent Living, 1619 Dayton Ave., St. Paul, MN 55104, 612/646-8342 (voice) 612/646-6048 (TDD). $9.00.

Describes a used equipment clearinghouse established and operated by the center. Provides information on how to set up a similar operation.

Walking: Funding Procedures. J. Kohn. Presented at a conference March 20, 1982, 4 pages. Available from author, Rehabilitation Engineering Center, Children's Hospital at Stanford, Palo Alto, CA.

Outlines procedures to procure funding for patients with mobility needs. Gives brief listing of funding agencies and of eligibility criteria.

"What's Left After Rowley? The Future of Advocacy in Special Education." K. Meador. *The Exceptional Parent*, February 1983, pages 59-64.

"What To Do When Health Insurance Won't Pay," P. Goodwin. *Better Homes and Gardens*. November 1987, pages 72-74.

Provides basic consumer information for dealing with rejected insurance claims.

"Wheelchair Manufacturers Discuss the Six-Point Plan." *Continuing Care*, July 1988, page 31.

Provides an overview of the new law governing Medicare reimbursement for home medical equipment and services, as it relates to wheelchairs. Effective 1/1/89, the law increased prevalance of rentals, probably promoting better quality products and services.

"When Insurer's Won't Pay Medical Bills," D. Rankin. *New York Times*. June 6, 1986.
Basic consumer information about ways to "fight back" when an insurance company balks at paying a claim or rescinds a policy. Stresses persistence.

"When Medicare Won't Pay," A. Berriman. *AOPA Almanac*. March 1985, pages 37-39.
Details instances when Medicare is considered a secondary source of payment instead of a primary source of payment.

"Who is Liable for Payment When Medicare Denies Coverages?" *Homecare*, August 1986, NAMES Resources section.

"Why Do They Do It?" P. Kraemer. *Homecare*, June 1986, pages 56-57.
Discusses dealer problems with reimbursement when unsupported equipment is provided; and, relates carrier wariness of computer-generated prescriptions because of some suppliers use of fictitious CMN forms.

Financing Adaptive Technology: A Guide to Sources and Strategies for Blind and Visually Inpaired Users. Steven Mendelsohn, May 1987, 206 pages. Available from: Smiling Interfaces, P.O. Box 2792, Church Street Station, New York, NY 10008-2792; $20.00; specify format: print, braille, audio cassette, Apple IIe disk. Also available through Demos Publications, 156 Fifth Avenue, Suite 108, New York, NY 10010. $24.95.
*Recommended. Although the guide focuses on the service systems and sensory aids which are of particular concern to visually disabled persons, everyone interested in rehabilitation technology should find it useful. Parallels to other disability groups are drawn, and similarities and differences in funding strategies are noted. Even if you are not involved with sensory aids or computer technology, if you are in the disability technology business, read this book.
In clear and practical language, the book delineates resources and describes procedures for paying for sensory aids. It explains most of the sources of technology funding: the vocational rehabilitation system, other programs of state agencies, the social security system, the tax system, the commercial credit system, government and nonprofit loan programs, veterans' benefits, the special education system, and more.
The guide explains the relevance and operation of each of these sources, analyzes issues and problems that arise in using them, suggests relationships among them, and alerts the equipment seeker to the complexities that may occur. The

guide aims at formulation of acquisition strategies, many of which are not commonly known to consumers or professionals.

Written by an attorney and rehabilitation practitioner, the material brings a unique perspective to the complicated and often poorly understood area of payment. The analysis of legislation related to adaptive technology policy is especially valuable, since it takes an advocates' approach of "if it doesn't say you can't, then you can" rather than the attitude most of the rest of us employ "if it doesn't say I can, then I can't." It encourages creativity in developing successful funding strategies. Each of the strategies reflects the personal experiences, the successes and the failures, of equipment seekers and service providers throughout the US. The guide is fully documented, with extensive legal, bibliographical and other resource information.

The major shortcoming of the document is its lack of analysis of the health care reimbursement system. (Sensory aids are not often reimbursed in medical systems.) If you are not already familiar with medical reimbursement processes, by reading only this book, you could easily overlook their importance for funding assistive technology. Since Medicare policy strongly influences medical/health reimbursement well beyond the Medicare system, it is imperative to have some understanding of Medicare's impact even if you never work with anyone eligible for Medicare.

[*This review was originally printed in the Summer 1987 RESNA newsletter "Assistive Technology Review."*]

T - #0195 - 101024 - C0 - 229/152/10 [12] - CB - 9781560240334 - Gloss Lamination